THE DISENCHANTED THERAPIST

S. J. SOUTHWELL

The Disenchanted Therapist

*Spot, navigate, and overcome
the common challenges of working as a therapist*

S. J. Southwell

Independent Publishing Network

Note to readers: Standards of clinical practice and protocol change over time, and no technique or recommendation is guaranteed to be safe or effective in all circumstances. This volume is intended as a general information resource for professionals practicing in the field of psychotherapy and mental health; it is not a substitute for appropriate training, peer review, and/or clinical supervision. Neither the publisher nor the author can guarantee the complete accuracy, efficacy, or appropriateness of any particular recommendation in every respect. The views expressed in this work are solely those of the author and do not necessarily reflect the views of the publisher, and the publisher hereby disclaims any responsibility for them.

Copyright © 2023 Sharon Southwell.

All rights reserved. No part of this book may be reproduced, stored, or transmitted by any means—whether auditory, graphic, mechanical, or electronic—without written permission of both publisher and author, except in the case of brief excerpts used in critical articles and reviews. Unauthorised reproduction of any part of this work is illegal and is punishable by law.

ISBN: 978-1-80352-343-9 (sc)
ISBN: 978-1-80352-344-6 (e)

Publisher: Independent Publishing Network
Publication date: July 17, 2023
Author: S. J. Southwell
Website: sharonsouthwellauthor.wordpress.com
Please direct all enquiries to the author.

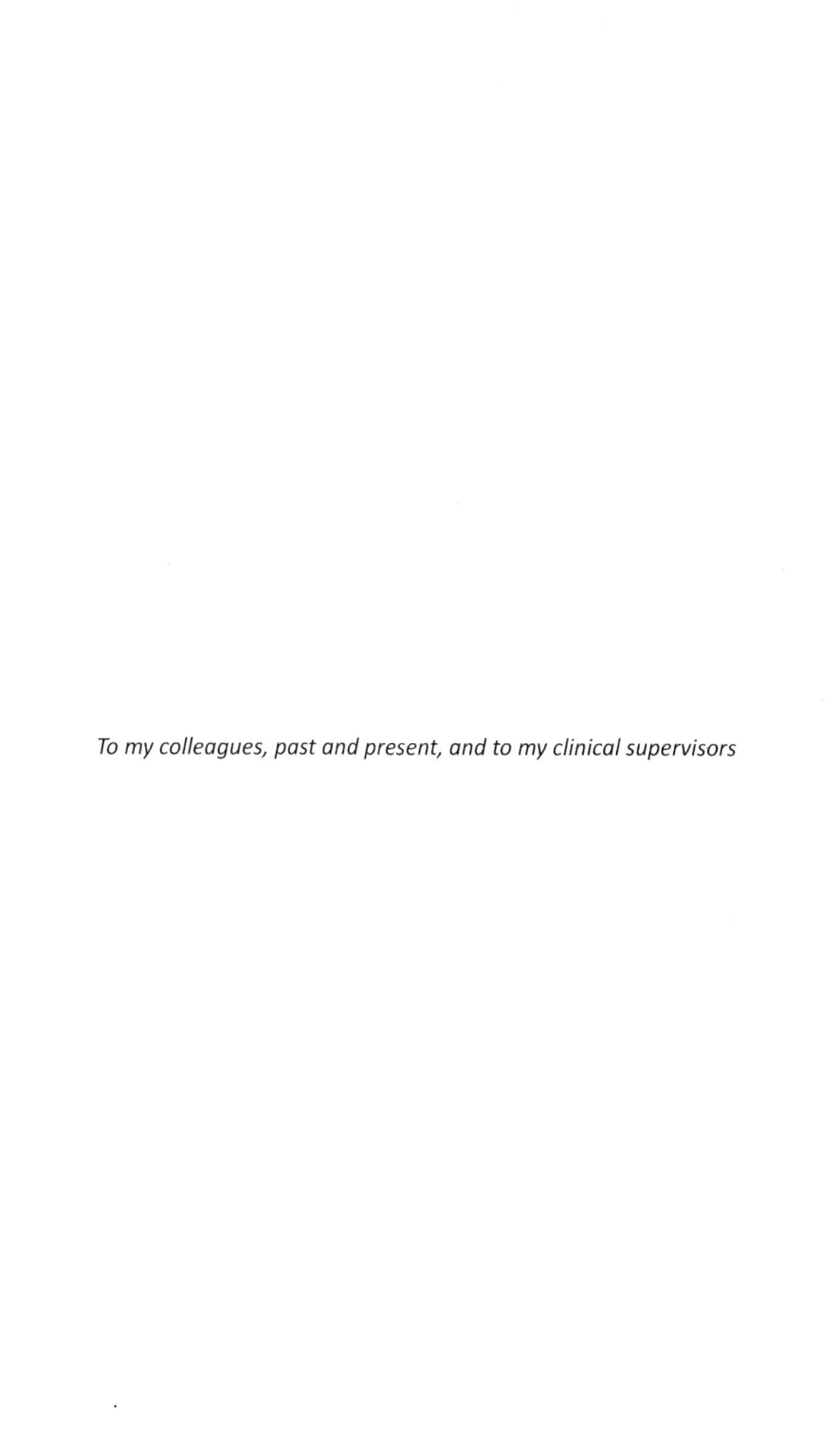

To my colleagues, past and present, and to my clinical supervisors

Acknowledgements

My clients, colleagues, and clinical supervisors have taught me so much about being a therapist. This book about the struggles of being a therapist and the ways through them would not exist without the many colleagues who have provided me wise counsel or clinical supervision. They include, Lindsay Gore, Patrick Newton, Sraddhanaya Hannan, Judi Brewster, the other supervisors at Quit Victoria, Kaaren Hawkes, Rebecca Diehm, Sue Murrant, Ross King, Marianne Weddell, Brendan Meagher, Jon Finch, Kirk Radcliff, Hugo Alarcon, Sandra Boughton, Mariavi Martinez, and Sean Harper. At just the right time, Gina Denholm provided experienced guidance about how to structure the fledgling manuscript. Many of its current merits reflect her advice while its infelicities remain my responsibility. Sandra Boughton and David Jones read an early version and provided encouragement. Finally, Vicki Grgic, Greg Restall, and Jenni Southwell brought their considerable capacities of heart and mind to the details and gaps in the final manuscript. I am deeply grateful to each of them.

Contents

Introduction 1

Chapter 1: *The Perfect Therapist and Other Traps,*
or Working With Our Habitual Thinking Patterns and Responses ... 8

    Our habitual thinking patterns and responses 9

        Unhelpful thinking habits 9

        Schemas, lifetraps, and defence mechanisms 11

    How these patterns affect our work.. 14

Chapter 2: *Know Yourself and Your History* 23

    Your background 23

    Your work history 25

    Your trauma history 26

    Attachment styles and personality traits..................................... 28

    Personal crises... 29

    Managing your physical and mental health 31

Chapter 3: *When the Work is Hard and Slow* 38

    Social disadvantage and multiple health issues 40

    Suggestions 41

    Clients behaving 'badly' 45

        Not turning up 45

        Anger 47

        Self-harm and suicidal behaviours... 49

    The compelled, the complainers, and the clients........................ 52

        The compelled 52

        The complainers 53

Complex cases 55
Clients who feel 'stuck' 55
Clients presenting in repeated crisis 57

Chapter 4: *Transference and Countertransference, Vicarious Trauma, and Moral Injury*.. 61

Transference and countertransference 62

Vicarious trauma 65

Moral injury... 71

Chapter 5: *Context is Everything* 77

Layers of context 78

Challenges and opportunities... 79

Chapter 6: *When Things Go to Hell in a Handbasket, or How to Handle Professional Crises* 89

Professional crises 89

Too much too soon, or 'Perhaps I'm not cut out for this work' ... 92

Is this burnout? 96

Chapter 7: *Crises of Faith* 104

Gratitude and appreciation 107

Follow-up research 108

Redefine your work and success 108

Hope and trust 109

Value what you do.. 110

Acceptance and grief.. 111

A change of heart 111

Recognising the spiritual dimension to your work 112

Chapter 8: *In Conclusion: Back to—Self-Care—Basics* 116
    Reflection 117
    Therapeutic strategies and skills 119
    Clinical supervision.. 119
    Professional development... 121
    Self-care... 122
Reference List..128

Introduction

Although I don't know you, as this book has caught your eye it is likely that you are a colleague, and probably a therapist, or someone who is concerned about the wellbeing of therapists. If you are a therapist then while it is possible that you picked up this book to prepare yourself better for your future career, or because you are concerned about the staff you supervise, the chances are that you are struggling in some way.

Therapy is tremendously rewarding work, both for what it can contribute to others and for what it can shape in us. At the same time though, because it requires authentic and committed engagement with others to support them in the business of change, it is extraordinarily demanding. We do this work in the context of our own patterns, histories, and responses, known or just as often, barely recognised or understood. The work needs to be created anew with each client but there are no guarantees of success. The hopes we have to be helpful often fall short with precisely the clients we know have suffered the most. We are routinely sitting with clients in deep distress and difficult circumstances, where we cannot help but be affected by the stories and emotions we encounter. There are innumerable practical and organisational constraints on what we can offer, matched only by the expectations from clients, our work places, and the community. When things go wrong, this can include the death of clients, professional sanction, or legal action. And all the while we do this work with imperfect tools and skills, and with varying degrees of scepticism and self-doubt, liabilities arising from our professional commitments to honesty and transparency in the face of discomfort.

Perhaps one or more of these challenges is weighing on you. You may be spending a lot of time talking to your colleagues and clinical supervisor about your concerns, or you may be avoiding them, aware of how negative your thoughts about your work, your clients, or therapy have become. You may have noticed persisting signs of stress, including impaired sleep, disturbed digestion, low and anxious mood, and avoiding tasks. You may have begun to wonder if your work is affecting your relationships with family and friends. Perhaps your colleagues or those close to you have told you they are concerned about you. Perhaps you are worried about whether therapy is the work for you. Perhaps the work is taking you to uncomfortable places. Perhaps you are wondering if therapy is effective or questioning whether you like people and working with them as much as you thought.

If you are struggling in these and other ways you are not alone. Each year, many previously committed therapists leave their work feeling discouraged and dispirited. You may have heard stories of therapists leaving their work or seen this happen to colleagues. Perhaps that is a real option for you as you begin to read this book. This problem afflicts the other caring professions as well, many of which have a significant turnover in the first years after training. Whether sooner in a career or later, the costs of such distress and associated decisions to leave the work are enormous for individuals, their careers, and their families. There are also significant costs for workplaces and work sectors that recruit and equip staff only to lose that investment in training.

I began my career in Australia. Prior to becoming a psychologist, I worked for 10 years in welfare and educational settings, supporting women and children affected by family violence, and later, university students. I have since worked as a psychologist for twenty years, providing assessment, counselling, and psychological treatment in a range of settings, including government services, not-for-profit health services, community health counselling services, and private practice.

I also worked as a health educator and trainer for a cancer support, prevention, and research institute, with a focus on encouraging preventative changes in health behaviours among populations with co-morbid mental health conditions. In addition, I worked initially as a counsellor and then as a supervisor and trainer of counsellors in a smoking cessation service, and as a trainer in a 24-hour volunteer-based counselling service.

Since moving into generalist psychological treatment and private practice in the last decade, I have worked with adults experiencing stress, depression, and anxiety conditions such as worry, social fearfulness, phobia, and panic attacks, as well as trauma, sleep difficulties, addictions, relationship and other interpersonal difficulties, and bereavement. The therapies I use include Cognitive Behaviour Therapy, Schema Therapy, Interpersonal Therapy, Motivational Interviewing to support behaviour change, Cognitive Processing Therapy to treat trauma, and mindfulness-based therapies including Acceptance and Commitment Therapy (ACT).

My clients have included individuals and families living with disability, individuals wanting to make changes to health behaviours, and adults seeking counselling and psychological treatment, across the age range, and from culturally and linguistically diverse backgrounds. At the time of writing this book, I find myself back in a university setting, but now in the UK, as a clinical supervisor for student-support staff and as a therapist for students.

I experienced elements of burnout in my late twenties when I was studying psychology and working full-time in a student-support role. I write about this experience in the section 'Is this burnout?', in Chapter 6. I recognised the experience for what it was because my professional training program covered the prevalence of burnout and the likelihood of psychologists leaving the profession. Having had that experience, I committed myself to doing whatever was necessary to prevent it ever happening again. Now such commitments can become a problem if they come with a degree of hypervigilance and reactivity to early signs of stress. Fortunately, that hasn't been the case for me. That said, over these 20 years, in order to keep my word to myself, I have changed jobs and work hours on several occasions. I have needed to regularly review my self-care plan, to increase the clinical supervision I am receiving, and to revisit how I am holding boundaries around my work. Periodically, I have needed to go deeper still, to reconsider what got me into therapy in the first place, whether that still matters to me, and how I want be present in the work going forward.

During my most recent period of professional dis-ease, I started writing about my experiences with therapist disenchantment as an exercise in reflection. I discovered something unexpected. I had fallen into, climbed out of, and recovered from many forms of therapist disenchantment. Over time I had become familiar with many of the risks of the work and had established personal and professional rules for myself about how to avoid them. As well as being encouraging, this review was also clarifying. It helped me recognise some of the many threads woven into my recent disenchantment but also how much I have learnt about doing therapy in a way that was good for my clients and for me. It also helped me identify the specific issues that were ailing me. Rather than one overwhelming mass of discontent, I could see the cause of the pain. When that was evident, I was able to prescribe my own remedies.

Soon into this writing, it occurred to me that other therapists might find it helpful to see written in one place something about the harder parts of being a therapist. Aside from a range of books about professional supervision and burnout, I have found it very difficult to locate candid books by therapists on this topic. I wonder if many of the things that motivate therapists to do their work, and many of the expectations that therapists and their workplaces and clients have of them, pose barriers for us in acknowledging these harder things we therapists know about our work. I very rarely hear colleagues talking about disenchantment, informally or in clinical supervision. I suspect that therapists who continue to struggle with some or more of these issues without support and resources eventually burnout, quietly or more spectacularly, or move sideways and perhaps even away from work with clients altogether.

This book is particularly for therapists who have been looking for help with distress, disappointment, dis-ease or disenchantment. In it I help therapists spot, navigate, and overcome the common emotional challenges of client work so that despite the occasional encounter with therapist disenchantment, they can continue to love the work, effectively support clients, and grow professionally and personally. It might be that having read this book you decide that a change is good and even needed, including perhaps a move away from this type of work. The aim of this book, however, is to support you in the possibility of continuing as a therapist, in one form or another.

When I use the words 'therapy' and 'therapist', I mean someone whose voluntary or paid work involves elements of counselling or 'talk therapy'. It is important to add that my experience with therapy has been largely in contexts of short- to medium-term work, in most instances where the timeframe and the nature of therapy reflect the limits of government or organisational funding models. Although I refer briefly to a range of psychodynamic ideas and concepts, a therapy field where long-term and open-ended therapy may still occur, much of what I have written here refers to the challenges and frustrations of time-limited and structured therapy. Even with this caveat in mind, the 'therapists' who might find this work relevant are a large group. They are counsellors and psychotherapists from all theoretical backgrounds. Along with therapists in private practice, they include psychiatrists, psychologists, social workers, clergy, pastoral workers, mentors, and coaches, working in a rich variety of roles and settings.

The stories I have included come from my own work or from the experiences of colleagues, or my work as a clinical supervisor or a therapist to therapists. To protect their identities all the stories from clients and therapists have been altered or are composites.

In this book I address many of the things that contribute to therapist disenchantment. They are grouped into three sections, the personal, practical, and professional, although these divisions are necessarily arbitrary and, in practice, there is tremendous crossover. The first section encourages you to reflect on different aspects of your life that affect your work as a therapist. These include your habitual thinking patterns and responses, in Chapter 1, and your personal history and current physical and mental health, in Chapter 2. The second section takes a look at what happens in the therapy space, especially when it is likely to affect the wellbeing of the therapist. This includes Chapter 3, which explores the situations in which therapy tends to be particularly hard or slow, and Chapter 4, on three ways in which client work can have particularly powerful and disturbing effects on therapists, transference and counter-transference, vicarious trauma, and moral injury. The final section addresses broader aspects of our professional experience, including our work context, in Chapter 5. The remaining chapters in this section address professional crises, including taking on too much client work too soon, and burnout, in Chapter 6, and professional crises of faith, in Chapter 7.

None of these sets of challenges stands in isolation, and all of them continue to be relevant over a career lifetime. My hope is that having mapped out the territory, you may avoid some of the risks, be better prepared than you might have been, and smile with recognition at those challenges you have survived.

With that focus on growth in mind, in each chapter I include 'Suggestions' for individual practitioners. Throughout, however, I am assuming that if you are having struggles in these areas, you have already set aside time to reflect on how your own thoughts and long-term ways of being in the world are contributing to the situation, and that you are intentionally using all the therapeutic strategies and skills you have available to support yourself. In addition, I am assuming that you are discussing your work with a professional, competent, and wise therapist-colleague who is acting as your clinical supervisor or peer mentor. Last but not least, I'm assuming that you are regularly planning and engaging in professional development learning that is relevant to the struggles you are experiencing, and that you are establishing a personal and professional discipline of intentional self-care.

It is, of course, much easier for me to write this list of essentials than it is for anyone to put them all in place. I urge you though, to make them your focus, and to return to and recover them whenever they become neglected. They are the basic foundation for addressing therapist disenchantment. Without them, you are building on shaky ground. They are so important that we return to them in the final chapter, Chapter 8, with some practical suggestions for how to consolidate your practice in these areas.

While this book primarily addresses individual therapists, one of the risks of that focus is the implication that each therapist is entirely responsible for their wellbeing in the workplace. In truth, many of the challenges that confront therapists arise out of workplace processes and cultures. With that in mind, the 'Recommendations' sections are followed by brief 'Workplace Tips' for managers of therapists or readers who are otherwise in a position to influence decisionmakers in their workplace.

Although the chapters have been written in a particular order and build on one another in the depth and complexity of the issues they address, they can also be read on their own. If you have come to this book with particular and pressing struggles and concerns, I encourage you to turn back to the Contents page, so you can see what speaks to you and dive in from there.

CHAPTER 1

The Perfect Therapist and Other Traps, or Working With Our Habitual Thinking Patterns and Responses

'I'm not sure than I can keep going,' Paul said, as he sat in my office. 'Every time I think about work, I feel all churned up ... and angry. There are too many cases for the staff to see, but our managers expect us to see them and follow all the processes and complete all the paperwork. They've lost touch with the pressures we are under ... if they ever were in touch. They don't have to sit in the room with such distress and such complicated problems, session after session. We are constantly being updated about changes to procedures. I've got to the point where I don't look at certain emails because if I do, I'll have to take time out that I don't have to change what I'm doing. I need to be answering calls from clients, or seeing them. It takes me all my time to do that, and I'm often working late, even though I try not to. The list of things to do is never-ending, but who else is going to follow-through for clients if I don't. That said, I suppose I could be more efficient. I'm just so tired and stressed it's hard to focus well. And I feel resentful about the time it takes from my family. I find it really hard to wind down when I get home. It's very easy to get into conversations with my partner about the day and my frustrations. She's very supportive but it's like she's expecting the day to be bad now, and I know that she worries about me. My sleep's been shocking. Also, I know the kids need me to be spending time with them and showing interest in their day as well. Really, I'm just glad they are watching TV or playing a game online when I get home, but I feel guilty about it all the same.'

This was how Paul introduced himself to me. As you read his description of his situation, perhaps you recognised some of your own thoughts or those you have heard from colleagues. Perhaps, with the benefit of some distance from Paul's situation and your therapist hat on you noticed what looked like themes. Perhaps you even wondered about his background and any long-term patterns that might be contributing to his choices in this situation. As therapists, our thinking patterns, core beliefs, schemas or longer-term thinking patterns, and our preferred defence mechanisms all affect our work with clients and how we think and feel about that work over the course of our careers. This chapter provides a brief introduction to these thinking and response patterns, how they affect our work, and some ways we can reflect on them more intentionally.

Our habitual thinking patterns and responses

Unhelpful thinking habits

Readers with a background in Cognitive Behaviour Therapy (CBT) will recognise the '10 unhelpful thinking patterns' that I've listed below. If they are new for you, you might want to mark the patterns that resonate with you as you read through the examples I've heard from therapists. Most people quickly identify these patterns in themselves and others, and can spot the ones they tend to use most. This is true of therapists as well as their clients.

1. All or nothing thinking

    My casenotes are bad.
    The management are hopeless (also a case of Labelling and mislabelling, see below).
    I need to be the perfect therapist.

2. Overgeneralisation

    When a medical referrer writes asking for more detailed reports: *I'm not good at writing reports.*
    I'm never going to find a job I want.
    After one or two bad experiences: *This place is terrible at paying staff properly.*

3. Mental filter

> After a seemingly positive session: *He looked flat. What was that about? He didn't tell me something important.*

4. Discounting the positive

> After a seemingly positive session: *I don't think I'm making much of a difference.*

5. Jumping to conclusions

    A. Mind-reading

    > *My boss doesn't like me. That's so unfair. I'm trying so hard.*
    > After a call to mental health emergency services about a client: *The responder thought I was exaggerating / out of my depth / didn't know what I was talking about. I need to be more persistent.*
    > After sharing a case with a seemingly supportive colleague, who offered a range of suggestions: *She doesn't think I made the right choice. She looked concerned. I won't go to her next time.*

    B. Fortune-telling

    > *That client is going to report me to the registration body. I will be in so much trouble if I get audited.*

6. Magnification or minimisation

    > *I'm way too emotional / thinking-preferenced / disorganised to be a therapist. I'm probably harming clients. Why did I become a therapist?*
    > 'You do an amazing job with your paperwork': *Isn't that what all of us are supposed to do?*

7. Emotional reasoning

    > *I'm exhausted. I'm not cut out for this work.*

8. "Should" statements

    > *I should be on top of e-mental health options for my clients. Our manager should know better.*

> *I ought to be better prepared for sessions.*
> *I have to return calls to client within (a given time frame).*
> *I must write those client reports this weekend.*
> *You've got to do your homework if you want to feel any better.*
> *My clients should work as hard as I do in therapy.*

9. Labelling and mislabelling

> *I'm a hopeless CBT / ACT / (your therapy of choice) therapist.*
> *He's entitled.*
> *She's a drama queen.*

10. Personalisation and blame

> *I'm responsible for his death.*
> *This is all his fault.*

Perhaps you spotted or have been reminded of some of your own unhelpful thoughts? If so, you are not alone. These are human thinking habits. Or perhaps you have heard some of these or variants from the lips of colleagues? This is an opportunity for you to make a mental or written note of your own examples of these thought patterns, whether longstanding or recent.

Schemas, lifetraps, and defence mechanisms

Often, our preferred thinking patterns arise from what CBT calls 'core beliefs' about ourselves, other people, and the world, and from more elaborate and long-term ways of seeing and being in the world, patterns that Schema Therapy, a close relative of CBT, labels 'schemas' or 'lifetraps'.

I'm thinking of a friend. She was in her early seventies at the time. She was not in a paid support role, but she was regularly ferrying people to doctors' appointments, delivering casseroles, helping people move, and making follow-up phone calls. She rarely brought attention to this activity but just kept at it. She was very reluctant to receive support herself and almost allergic to having people help her. She had serious chronic health issues of her own, which she mostly sought to downplay. Just occasionally, when very tired or at times when her own health issues were debilitating, she would speak irritably about people not present and their lack of care to her. Just occasionally, when someone suggested she was being a bit smothering, she would be hurt and angry. We will return to my friend in a moment.

Schema Therapy provides one of many therapy models for thinking about our long-term patterns. It posits that patterns like these are shaped during childhood, as a result of both common-and-garden and more grievous gaps in parenting and nurture. For at least some of us, they are then reinforced by later experiences. While many people in the non-patient population may not endorse any of these patterns at a level that significantly affects their functioning, most of us recognise one or more of these tendencies:

- The schemas that are related to *disconnection and rejection* include abandonment/instability, mistrust/abuse, emotional deprivation (with the subsets of deprivation of nurturance, empathy, and protection), defectiveness/shame, and social isolation/alienation.

- Those related to *impaired autonomy and performance* include dependence/ incompetence, vulnerability to harm or illness, enmeshment/underdeveloped self, and failure.

- Those related to *impaired limits* include entitlement/grandiosity, and insufficient self-control/self-discipline.

- Those related to *other-directedness* are subjugation (including subjugation of needs and of emotions), self-sacrifice, and approval-seeking/recognition seeking.

- Finally, those related to *over vigilance and inhibition* include negativity/pessimism, emotional inhibition, unrelenting standards/hyper-criticalness, and punitiveness.

Schema Therapy suggests that much of the time a person with such a pattern will completely 'surrender' to it. For example, someone with a self-sacrifice schema may feel compelled to be helpful and solicitous. At other times, often under considerable pressure, they will flip to what looks like the opposite behaviour, the 'counter-attack,' which might include demanding and angry responses when unappreciated. At other times still, they may behave in ways that 'avoid' the pull and pressure of this self-sacrificing pattern, turning off the phone, avoiding clinical or management supervision, dropping out of social commitments, or over-indulging in one form of self-soothing behaviour or another. Schema Therapy refers to these three patterns, surrender, counter-attack, and avoidance, as 'maladaptive coping strategies.' Much of the work of this therapy is helping people to understand at a deep emotional level the origins of these patterns and how they currently operate in their lives. With this understanding, recognising that these patterns—forged as ways of surviving in childhood—may not be serving them as well as adults, they may be more able to consider change.

As you look at those patterns, I wonder if any remind you of clients, relatives, or yourself? Thinking back to my friend's story, perhaps you know someone who has a long-term way of being in the world that sounds familiar? I have written this story to emphasise my friend's 'self-sacrificing' pattern. She has a strong dose of unrelenting standards / hyper-criticalness as well, which is a common combination for therapists, when sprinkled with a dash of 'emotional deprivation.' By a sprinkle of 'emotional deprivation', I mean the many related patterns that adults exhibit when they experienced some degree of deprivation as a child, be this of nurturance, empathy, or protection. Very often, young children, who have no choice but to accept this situation, respond with a pattern of seeming early competence and independence, including being helpful and caring to others, all still with an unconscious longing that this independence and competence will be admired and win them the emotional care that feels lacking.

Readers who are familiar with psychodynamic therapies will recognise in these 'maladaptive coping strategies' features of defence mechanisms. These are automatic behaviours that we use to ward off anxiety and to limit how much we are aware of and disturbed by the possibility of actual dangers or stressors, within and without. There are many defence mechanisms, some more adaptive than others. They range from altruism, humour, and sublimation, to dissociation, intellectualisation, and repression, to devaluation or idealisation, denial, and projection, to autistic fantasy, acting-out and passive-aggression, and at the extremes, to delusional projection, psychotic denial, and psychotic distortion. For our purposes, the important point is that we all have defence mechanisms we use frequently. Under pressure, at least occasionally, most of us find ourselves using some of the less adaptive mechanisms as well.

How these patterns affect our work

Our thinking patterns, schemas and defence mechanisms affect our work with clients in many ways. Here are four of them.

To begin with, these patterns are shaped by the same things that contribute eventually to our motivations for becoming therapists, our particular life histories. As Louis Cozolino points out in his book, *The Making of a Therapist: A practical guide for the inner journey* (2004), therapists often have a role as peacemakers or counsellors in their families of origin, and there is as well a broad cultural expectation that women, in particular, will be there for others. If being helpful was an effective way of being in the world for you as a child, or if a generally self-sacrificing way of being in the world was modelled to you by one or both parents, there is an increased likelihood that a career that involves helping others will appeal to you. It will feel familiar and in keeping with what has already become a long-term way of being in the world. Knowing what schemas contribute to the strength of your motivation to provide therapy is important because the challenges of therapy will almost inevitably cause you to question your motivations. It can help to have a sense of what brought you to your choice in the first place. Perhaps, once you know in a clear-eyed way what brought you to the work, you may decide you no longer need to do this work, or you may commit yourself to it anew and with a more nuanced conviction.

We will return to the importance of our histories in the second chapter. The two areas, though—our thinking patterns and our histories—always interact. As an example, our thinking patterns, schemas, and defence mechanisms shape the way we see the world and respond to events. To be more specific, when unexamined, they may limit the choices we feel we have available, throwing us almost unconsciously into particular unhelpful behaviours. For example, and using language from Schema Therapy, a therapist with a self-sacrificing pattern may find it very hard to be appropriately assertive. Like many of our clients, we may need to learn and then practice assertiveness skills, again and again. Successful work as a therapist requires that you can draw on many strategies, flexibly. For example, this might include being able to be permitting and collaborative in some situations, and then when risk or safety issues are present, being able to take up your authority as a leader in the relationship and be appropriately assertive about the focus of the session or the consequences of particular choices by the client.

Let's extend out this idea about the ways schemas can limit our choices and the benefits of growing in flexibility around our schemas. Most of us have at least one or two active schema areas and some of us will have more. Sometimes there are tensions among them. Under pressure, people with some impulsivity in the mix may find it hard to organise their lives sufficiently to run a private practice. To meet the needs of their clients and business, they may have to focus on acquiring particular disciplines that might otherwise feel irksome. For therapists with some entitlement or approval-seeking in the mix, the often-anonymous work of day-to-day therapy may feel unrewarding. Unless they can find some ways of reframing the work to themselves, they may want to look for more high-profile roles or more prestigious clientele. Similarly, if unaware, therapists with a sense of vulnerability to harm or a tendency to negativity and pessimism, may find themselves at risk of anxiety or low mood, when they encounter challenges within the workplace. The flexibility needed in each of these instances can emerge from a combination of awareness, recognising the need to change, and a willingness to try new things.

As you might expect from the examples above, our schemas also affect the way we will tolerate clients who don't get better quickly or who behave in challenging ways. Even the most caring therapist is capable of anger and of bullying or punitive words or actions, however much they will soon regret them. A very common counter-attack to self-sacrifice is anger, when a person feels they have been pushed beyond what is reasonable. If you don't have effective assertiveness skills in place, your client and the therapy might be at risk in this situation. Similarly, a common counter-attack to unrelenting standards / hyper-criticalness—also known as 'high standards' or perfectionism—is to 'drop the ball' or to push back and say, 'I can't do it anymore'. Mostly this is momentary and not a problem, but sometimes this means we don't follow through on promises made to clients. Similarly, therapists with high standards, or some defectiveness or failure in the mix, may find themselves, on the one hand, having negative thoughts about themselves as therapists, or alternatively redoubling their efforts, and trying to spur their clients on, potentially in ways that leave clients feeling inadequate or pressured.

As hinted at above, our longer-term patterns also affect our ability to tolerate that package Louis Cozolino describes of sitting with not knowing, being human, 'being slight crazy,' and not having it all together as a person. If you have perfectionistic tendencies, high standards, or imposter syndrome, acknowledging frailty is hard and can easily lead to over-striving. Also, it takes time to grow. We can't simply will it. We need it to be a continuing commitment. However difficult this is, remember that if it is hard for you to sit with your own slow process of change, this will necessarily affect how hard it is for you to sit with the slow process of change in others. Said positively, the more you are able to tolerate your own frailty and struggles, the better you will be able to do this for others. Indeed, the more compassion you can generate for yourself in this process, the more likely it is that you will be able to model this to clients.

Finally, our long-term patterns affect our ability to reach, hold, and return to something like a balance between the different parts of our life: our family, community, work, recreational, self-care, and spiritual commitments. This balance is always under tension and our schemas add to the push and pull, pushing us, for example, towards taking on more responsibility, or pulling us towards excessive, emotionally-detached self-soothing, be this with screen-time, substances, or shopping. Please feel free to insert here your preferred 'avoiding' distractions. When the balance in our lives is under this sort of pressure, it often adds to or worsens our sense of depletion, where we are giving out too much, and not receiving sufficient in return.

You will notice that as we acknowledge these impacts of our thinking habits and long-term patterns, this almost immediately points us to both the importance of becoming aware of our patterns and the areas where we might make change.

Now while some therapist trainee-programs expect that students will undergo their own therapy or analysis, many therapists reach client work with limited experience of self-reflection, let alone any in-depth understanding of their own patterns. Not having completed considerable self-reflection in our training, for many of us the pressures of our work pose ongoing barriers in deepening our awareness of our own patterns. Unfortunately, there are huge risks for practitioners who try to do therapeutic work with client without growing deeper in their knowledge of themselves and their ability to work with that content. We need more than self-care, as it is often superficially defined. We need to continue to grow in our knowledge of ourselves.

Suggestions

Here are some suggestions for how to begin to work with your habitual thinking patterns and responses, particularly if you suspect they may be contributing to your experience of therapist disenchantment.

Thinking habits

We start here with some of the most foundational practices, ones that many of us routinely share with our own clients. If you have never done so before, consider the '10 unhelpful thinking habits' for yourself. You might look back at the brief listing early in this chapter. Descriptions for these thinking patterns are also available online and in David Burns's *The Feeling Good Handbook*. Which do you recognise in yourself, and which are most habitual? Have you noticed any in operation in your work as a therapist? As you have picked up this book, I suspect that your answer will be 'yes'. If not though, take some time to reflect on that question. You might list some of the most familiar, long-standing, recent, or pressing work-related negative and anxious thoughts you notice. You might think back to Paul's opening words to me and consider what you might say about your work experience right now.

Once you have a list of your most compelling thoughts, the next invitation is to see if there are any that can be dispelled through some gentle but clear-eyed evaluation and challenge. Please use whatever therapeutic skills you have available to engage with such thoughts, attitudes, and beliefs about your work. This might even be material for some professional development journaling or conversations with your clinical supervisor.

To help you with this process of evaluation, I have included below a list of ways of evaluating what CBT calls 'automatic' negative and anxious thoughts and underlying rules and assumptions. I'd invite you to read through the list and mark or highlight the questions that you think would help you to evaluate, reconsider, or get some perspective on your regular work-related negative and anxious thoughts:

Is it a true fact? Is what I am thinking or feeling verifiably true?
What evidence do I have for this thought? What is the evidence that supports this thought?
What is the evidence against this idea?
Am I jumping to conclusions?
Am I confusing a thought with a fact?
Is there any alternative way of looking at this situation? Is there any alternative explanation?
Am I assuming that my view of things is the only one possible?
How would someone else think about this situation?
Are my judgments based on how I feel, rather than what is actually happening?
Am I setting myself unrealistic or unobtainable standards?
Am I forgetting relevant facts or over-focusing on irrelevant facts?
Am I thinking in all or nothing terms?
Am I overestimating how responsible I am for the way things work out?
Am I overestimating how much control I have over how things turn out?
Am I only paying attention to the black side of things?
Am I overestimating the chances of disaster?
Am I exaggerating the importance of events?

What would happen? What would be so bad about that?
What's the worst that could happen? Could I live through it?
What is the best that could happen?
What is the most realistic outcome?
How will things be in X months or a year's time?
Am I overestimating how likely the event is?
Am I worrying about the way things ought to be, instead of accepting and dealing with them as they are?
Am I underestimating what I can do to deal with the problem/situation?
Am I assuming that I can do nothing to change my situation?
Am I predicting the future instead of experimenting with it?
Is this a familiar 'old' story that my mind has brought out again to string me along?
Even if my thought is true, is it helpful to me?
What is the effect of me believing the automatic thought?
Do negative thoughts help or hinder me?
What could be the effect of changing my thinking?
Are there any benefits to me in buying into this thought?
What thinking errors might I be making?
Am I asking questions that have no answers?
Am I using ultimatum words in my thinking, like 'always,' 'never,' 'everyone,' 'no one,' 'everything,' and 'nothing'?
Am I condemning myself as a total person on the basis of a single event?
Am I concentrating on my weaknesses and forgetting my strengths?
Am I blaming myself for something which is not really my fault?
Am I taking things personally which have little or nothing to do with me?
Am I expecting myself to be perfect?
Am I using a double standard, expecting more of myself than I would of someone else?
Does holding on to the thought or attitude serve my best interests? Does it make me happy, calm, peaceful, and fulfilled?
Are my thoughts and attitudes advancing and protecting my health?
Do my thoughts about myself push me into situations that put my well-being at risk?
Does this attitude or belief get me more of what I want, need, and deserve? Or is it leading me toward or keeping me in circumstances that I don't want?

Having encouraged you to engage in evaluation of your thoughts, do keep in mind that one or more of the studies looking at the effectiveness of elements of Acceptance and Commitment Therapy (ACT) suggest that evaluation and challenging may be less important than simply noticing the pattern. *Noticing* itself may be sufficient to help us 'defuse' from a thought, its emotional impact, and the power that it might have had to drive our behaviours.

Schemas and longer-term patterns

If you don't already have some framework for thinking about your long-term thinking patterns, consider how you might find one.

You might read the two almost-official self-help books for Schema Therapy, *Reinventing Your Life: The breakthrough program to end negative behaviour and feel great again* (1994) by Jeffrey E. Young and Janet S. Klosko, and—if you find that you have a reasonable number of schemas—*Breaking Negative Thinking Patterns: A Schema Therapy self-help and support book* (2015), by Gitta Jacob, Hannie van Genderen and Laura Seebauer.

Alternatively, if your clinical supervisor is familiar with schemas or defence mechanisms, they may be able to assist you with some assessment and facilitate conversations about how these patterns are relevant for your work. While psychodynamically-influenced clinical supervision moves more readily into this territory, it is often a new experience for therapists who are used to conventional clinical supervision that focusses largely on the client and only briefly on therapist responses. You and your clinical supervisor may need to clarify those boundaries and how to keep these discussions focussed on your work, thereby distinguishing clinical supervision from therapy. Having a model for your supervision can help in this regard. For example, the seven-eyed model from Peter Hawkins and Robin Shohet, in *Supervision in the Helping Professions* (2006), provides a framework for thinking about client-therapist work, therapist responses, the therapist-supervisor contribution to the picture, and the broader context as well.

If you are already seeing a therapist who is familiar with Schema Therapy, or you are open to finding one, some sessions exploring this territory would be a worthwhile investment. If you have patterns that you recognise are persistently troublesome, perhaps a few more sessions might be useful.

If your clinical supervisor can't help and some brief therapy doesn't seem manageable, perhaps one of your colleagues who uses Schema Therapy might be willing to provide you an assessment and feedback, particularly if they can claim some hours of professional development in the process.

It might even be that having read this chapter you decide to commence or re-commenced some therapy yourself.

Workplace Tip

If you are in a position to influence decision-making in your workplace, do what you can to introduce, support, and nurture the active use of clinical supervision among client-facing staff.

Take-home message:

To continue as a therapist, you will need to address the challenges posed not only by the work but by your habitual ways of being in the world. The better you know your own thought patterns and the more practice you have noticing and modifying your patterns—when you recognise this is needed—the more flexibility you will have in your choices, especially when you encounter the harder aspects of work and life.

Where to next?

If you have been a therapist for a while, you may be thinking that this brief introduction to thinking patterns, schemas, and defence mechanisms is only scratching the surface of your concerns or disenchantment. If that's you, then be assured that we are laying a necessary foundation for more reflection on your own processes and for a thorough exploration of the range of external pressures that intersect with them. In the next chapter we take a deeper look at how our personal histories, current experiences, and health affect our work.

Chapter 2

Know Yourself and Your History

My colleague Rita migrated from South America. She told me that when she first arrived in Australia without her family she felt very lonely. She noticed that suburban streets were empty most of the day, as though the community had vanished. This was a huge contrast to life back home where people constantly stopped to chat on the path and outside shops and children were ever-present, playing in the street. This was a big adjustment for Rita and one of the reasons she worked to bring out her family. It also helped her to appreciate the loneliness felt by so many of our clients: 'I'm always listening out for their connections or lack of them,' she told me. Rita's story illustrates some of the very many aspects of our personal histories that have an impact on our values and the way we work as therapists.

Having begun to reflect on what we bring to therapy and our lives as therapists through our thinking patterns, let's look both backward and forward: back to the history that shaped those thinking patterns in the first place, including our personal background, work history, trauma history, and attachment styles and personality traits, and then forward to our current experiences, recent crises, and the mental and physical health conditions that we are juggling.

Your background

What aspects of your story have deeply shaped your views and attitudes? These experiences may not have been 'traumatic', but if they have shaped strong views about you and others and the world, they will be relevant to your work as a therapist. I'm thinking here about whether you are a man or woman, transgender or non-binary, and how family, community, and broader cultural attitudes to gender have affected your life. And how do you think of your sexual orientation and how attitudes to sexual orientation have affected your life? I'm also thinking about your ethnic and socio-economic background, what communities you grew up in, and about any stories of migration told by your family. Have you been on the receiving end of harassment, discrimination, or prejudice? Did you grow up in communities where groups other than yours were harassed or discriminated against? Did you or your family experience successes or setbacks? What stories did they tell about themselves? What was your family structure and general tone? What roles did you have in that family? What is the shape of your current family? What roles do you have? Do you now care for children, elderly relatives, or relatives with mental or physical disabilities? How are those relationships? Do you have a disability yourself? How is that experience for you and what do you bring to it from the attitudes of your community and family of origin?

These and many other aspects of our histories shape who we are as therapists and how we think about and respond to our clients, both those who seem to have very different histories from our own, and those with apparently similar stories. Where there are commonalities, such stories may help with our empathy and even our knowledge of resources, as well as informing our commitment to seek for justice on behalf of our clients. On the other hand, such commonalities may also make it harder for us to see both the details and the bigger picture of a client's life, where their stories diverge from our own.

While we are talking about our personal histories, I invite you to consider your relationships with your parents or early primary caregivers. Are your parents living or dead? What is or was your relationship like? Have you done enough reflective work on those relationships? What parenting styles did you experience? Were one or both strict and sergeant-major-like, with elements of authoritarianism, or more coach-like or authoritative, or absent or permissive, or a combination? Did or do you have a reasonably easy relationship with your parents, an enmeshed and dependent one, or a distant, conflictual or adversarial one? These experiences affect both how we interact with clients and how we interact with colleagues, bosses, and organisations. I would encourage you to reflect on your work history and how you have interacted with leaders. Are there any patterns? As we will explore in Chapter 5, workplace dynamics also affect how we function as therapists. It can help to be alert to this aspect of your history that might pull you in particular ways in your interaction with leaders, or shape your own leadership style as this is expressed in your role as a colleague, supervisor, and therapist.

Your work history

In thinking about your history, consider also where you have worked and how that work has shaped you. As with the other parts of our history, these experiences can have a significant impact on our work as therapists, for good or ill.

As an example, while I was still an undergraduate, I worked in a women's refuge over several summers and eventually part-time. This was a formative experience. As a result, in the world of therapy that can often be permissive, this is an area where I feel most confident expressing categorical values. Whenever a client acknowledges receiving or committing violence, I clearly, firmly, and respectfully, name this as utterly unacceptable and criminal. I offer support for those who have experienced abuse. I urge clients who acknowledge violence to embrace non-violence and to begin by drawing a line in their relationships, ruling out emotional abuse or physical violence. Similarly, when a woman—it is usually a woman—comes to see me for help to think differently about her abusive partner or for help to better handle the symptoms of anxiety and depression arising from abusive relationship dynamics, I am clear that while I will do what I can to support her to reflect on or change her situation, I will not use the tools of therapy to patch her up so that she can return to the relationship without her partner being held accountable. I have never had a client object to either intervention, although I'm aware that both are confronting. I believe that in these respects my experiences have shaped in me a clarity that is needed on such topics. At the same time, though, I'm committed to working with clients where they are.

By contrast and continuity, however, I have experienced considerable difficulty providing therapy to violent men who are ambivalent about their behaviour. These men rarely attend private practice voluntarily. The ones that come to mind were sent by local corrections services. In most instances I have asked male colleagues to take on these cases, instead. I know that it is very hard for me to hear these clients well, in a way that might inform skilful action from me and open the way for these men to consider change. In these circumstances, it seems most ethical to admit my limitations and to support these clients to transfer to another therapist.

Your trauma history

My client was a young police officer, Gary. He had grown up in a household where domestic violence was present, and in a community where violence was more common than in the general population. This was a reason he decided to become an officer. He wanted to help. After training, Gary was placed at a station in a neighbouring suburb to the one where he grew up. Day after day he was taking calls out to deal with family and other violence. He was good at the work, but it was highly stressful, and the need was seemingly never ending. In truth, all that his unit were doing was patching people up, processing their apprehended violence and restraining orders through the courts, and repeating the process. Although the team were making a positive difference to individual families, the root causes of the violence were not being addressed. Gary's history unexpectedly became a liability. He began to notice himself having hopeless thoughts about the prevalence of violence. Very quickly he came to dread the work. This was made harder by some conflict with a more senior staff member. He began to find himself feeling quite emotional at inconvenient times, and having significant anxiety symptoms. He began to doubt his calling to policing. This came with a certain despair when he considered all the effort he had gone through to get to this point. You may recognise that Gary was spiralling into burnout. He held himself back from this by identifying a glimmer of hope. With some extra experience he would be eligible to apply for a type of community policing that involved proactive programs of one sort or another.

> *There, he hoped, he could actually make a difference.*

Although Gary is not a therapist, his story highlights the ways that our backgrounds and trauma histories can complicate our experiences of caring work with others and contribute to professional distress and disenchantment.

A few years ago, I was presenting a case to my clinical supervisor where my client had experienced domestic violence. At some point, unexpectedly, she asked me, 'Have you experienced domestic or intimate partner violence or some other significant interpersonal trauma yourself?' I was taken aback but immediately understood the reason for her question. I was taken aback because my experience of clinical supervision has touched only superficially on my own life story. I suspect that I'm not alone in that experience, and that this gap in supervision occurs because both clinical supervisors and supervisees generally want to avoid anything that looks like therapy. That said, the life, person, and body of the therapist is very clearly affected by and active in the process of therapy, and there are so many ways in which these topics might be relevant to clinical supervision.

In this instance, my clinical supervisor, who had been a clinical psychologist for forty years, knew what she was doing. There is something about severe traumas and particularly the life-threatening ones that enable them to lodge powerfully in our emotion memories. These emotion memories can be readily triggered by life-threatening content described by clients. As well as producing strong emotional responses, traumatic experiences are often very formative. We develop stories about ourselves, the world, and other people around such experiences, and those stories can be quick to come to our mind and our lips when we encounter someone telling a somewhat related story. The challenge here is to avoid the temptation to make the therapy session about you. It might be, of course, that this shared experience will aid your empathy and therapeutic presence. There is just the risk, though, that it will be harder for you to hear your client's journey, responses, and meaning-making, which might be quite different from your own.

For some therapists, in their choice of clients, there is a form of trauma re-enactment going on, where they are placing themselves back in contexts like the one in which they grew up, because they are familiar. For others, this is as well a form of 'trauma mastery,' an unconscious attempt to somehow overcome as an adult and in a skilled way the challenges that were insurmountable in childhood. Most of us are not conscious of these reasons for our professional choices when we start out as therapists. Largely unconscious, those motivations can add a drive to our work and fuel our motivation and effectiveness, but they can also readily tilt us towards places of imbalance in our work, and especially toward inadequate self-care.

Attachment styles and personality traits

Let's take this one step further, combining what you have reflected on so far about your own thinking patterns and history. What do you know about your own attachment style? Over many years of attending and participating in church communities, I have observed patterns in how people engage with new and incoming pastors, the leaders of the church, and possible 'parent-figures' of the community. While how this looks is also affected by the style of the incoming leader and their gender and age in relation to congregation members, I have noticed subtle but consistent patterns of confidence and security, helpfulness, reliability, co-operation, ingratiation, seduction, defiance, complaint, fear, and distancing. How about you? Have you noticed similar patterns in others or yourself? What do you know about your attachment patterns? Do you generally fall into the more securely attached, the more anxious, or avoidant patterns, or are there even elements of disorganised attachment in your experience?

Knowing about attachment styles is important for your work with clients in at least four ways. First, it may help you to be alert to their styles and how they affect their interactions with others, including you. Second, your behaviour will affect your clients and to some extent this will be related to their attachment styles. If you place limits on your client that they experience as rejecting or abandoning, this may trigger a habitual anxious or distancing response from them. When you are alert to such possibilities you can work with the responses rather than reacting to them. Third, you may find your own attachment patterns triggered when established clients don't turn up or keep you at arm's length or die. Finally, your attachment patterns may influence how events in the workplace and among colleagues affect you. To be specific, repeatedly across my career I have noticed that the ways that colleagues respond to a change of leadership or structure vary tremendously but consistently. I have come to suspect that this is often related to a factor that is invisible and generally not discussed among therapists: our attachment styles.

Finally, what do you know about your general personality structure? There is a range of models and assessment tools available. One well-regarded theory of personality is that of the Big Five Personality dimensions: extraversion, agreeableness, openness, conscientiousness, and neuroticism. As you might imagine, your personality profile will make a difference to the general ways in which you interact with others. It will also affect the ways you respond to and think about clients and colleagues with very different personalities to your own. Imagine, for example, how a somewhat anxious, conscientious and agreeable colleague and a somewhat laidback, occasionally argumentative, and not particularly conscientious colleague might experience or view each other. It is very easy to make negative judgments about someone whose stable personality structure is markedly different from your own on several dimensions. Their behaviour may often seem inexplicable or deficient. We may need to remind ourselves that personality structures, ours included, are largely created by forces outside of our control including genes and early nurturing.

Personal crises

When I worked at Lifeline, a free 24-hour support-line, the Australian version of UK-based Samaritans, on the team training volunteers for their role as telephone counsellors, the application form asked people if they had experienced a bereavement, traumatic event, or mental health condition in the last two years. The aim of this question was not to screen out applicants but instead to highlight them to the training team. When their applications were otherwise promising, we called applicants to ask a little more about their backgrounds. We also shared with them our observations in working with trainees that recent experiences were often fresher and more impactful and more likely to be triggered by similar content in counselling calls. We normalised such responses but said that we had a duty of care to trainee-counsellors not to enrol them into the course if it was too early in their healing journey. Just occasionally, otherwise successful applicants decided to defer their enrolment to our next intake. The vast majority went into the course somewhat prepared and knowing that we were available for support if needed.

My experience with Lifeline points to an extension of the idea that we should know our histories. Recent events occurring in our personal and work lives have an impact on our work. The whole of life happens to therapists during their work. A colleague's spouse died. Others have become carers to family members with disabilities and to elderly relatives. Many colleagues have become parents for the first time. It is very hard before such life events to have a sense of the impact they will have on your work. In my experience observing many female colleagues planning for their first child, perhaps one had a realistic sense of how all-consuming the experience would be. Similarly, I have routinely observed parents expecting a second child thinking that this will be much less of an adjustment than having the first one. Most quickly discover their home workload more than doubles.

The arrival of an additional child is a fine example of how the usual stuff of life, things we wouldn't even call 'crises,' affect us and have a potential to affect our work with clients: illness, family dramas and conflict, and all the normal parts of parenting, to name a few.

Changes in our lives, including major life changes, come with stress. As example, two of the most stressful events in life are getting married and moving house. While often generally positive experiences, both involve large amounts of change. This is true of other major life changes as well. When life changes in these ways, we may be stressed, tired, preoccupied, or grieving, even as we continue to provide support to others. We may find ourselves having stronger emotional reactions than usual to particular client stories, or being more likely to share our own stories, or to give advice out of our own stories. While the impact on clients may be minimal, sometimes it isn't. We are each responsible for noticing the impact of such life events on our work and taking steps to care for ourselves and keep our work safe and effective.

Managing your physical and mental health

How we look after ourselves at times of stress and crisis is a natural bridge between self-management of our inner patterns and responses and self-management of our physical and mental health. Thinking about the impact of health conditions on our work, I am reminded of a colleague with severe chronic migraines who was regularly unable to attend scheduled appointments with clients. The administrative staff were constantly rescheduling her sessions. Eventually—and unfortunately, given her skill and experience— without a self-management and workplace plan in place, she was not able to continue in the role.

Her story reminds me of a colleague with a very different set of challenges. I read about him in one of my professional organisation's publications. A therapist in the later stages of his career, he had received a diagnosis of dementia. He knew that he could possibly work for several years more and he had clients who wanted to continue therapy with him. He knew that some of the challenges of dementia would include increased forgetfulness, difficulties with organisation, and eventually, diminished insight into his own difficulties. Together with trusted and wise colleagues, he devised a plan where his functioning would be monitored and supported. The aim of the plan was to enable him to continue his work as long as it was possible, while providing responsible care for his clients.

This is an impressive example of the sort of planning that I would encourage you to consider for any physical and mental health issues you are aware of or that emerge during your work as a therapist. Given the incidence and prevalence of depression and anxiety in the community, a fair proportion of therapists are experiencing one of these conditions at any given time, and even more have experienced such conditions and may be at increased risk of a further episode. A smaller number will have one of the less common major mental illnesses, including the bi-polar and psychotic disorders. Similarly, some proportion of therapists will have traits of personality disorders and a larger proportion will have either current or past difficulties with substances and other addictive patterns. It doesn't take much imagination, in any of these cases, to see how these conditions might affect your work as a therapist.

Most therapists, like their medical colleagues, are nervous about reporting their mental health struggles and diagnoses to clinical or management supervisors or professional bodies, fearing negative judgement and a corresponding impact on their job security or career progression. This is understandable. That said, in increasing numbers, professions and communities are expressing through regulations and legislation their recognition that terminating a person's employment based on their mental health condition, a recognised disability, is discrimination. In some places workplace training is now available about how to effectively support and manage the mental health of employees. Such changes assume that it is in fact the responsibility of the workplace to enable staff members with a disability to complete their work. As well, many professional bodies are trying to build into their processes the understanding that it is a positive step for professionals to disclose mental health conditions, rather than something to be penalised. If something is disclosed, it may increase the chances that it can be managed and that the staff member can be cared for and retained, functioning well and safely themselves and as a contributing and effective member of the team. It is true, of course, that legislation and policy often lead the way, with practice remaining somewhat patchy and delayed, so use your best judgement about any disclosures, but please prioritise your self-care and safe work.

Suggestions

One way to deepen your appreciation of the links between your history in all its aspects, the various elements of your personality, recent challenging experiences and crises, and your work as a therapist, is to commit to a process of reflection, where you attempt to be mindful of the circumstances where you have stronger responses than normal, or responses that later seem to you unwarranted or surprising. Consider writing about your observations and reflections and bringing them to your clinical supervision.

Your background

This may be a new area of reflection for you, or one to which you are returning because you have begun to suspect that your history is contributing to your distress at work. Consider journalling in response to the questions I asked earlier, about your background. Perhaps, just as we might do this for a client, you might write out a genogram for yourself, reflecting on the way your family history shapes your attitudes to work. Keep in mind both the positive ways in which your background may have affected you and shaped your motivation for working as a therapist, and the aspects of your background that might constitute vulnerabilities for you. It is possible that, like Gary, the two are closely related for you.

Reflect on your work history and how you have interacted with leaders. Are there any patterns? Do those patterns appear to relate in any ways to the relationships you had to early care-givers? You might consider taking parenting or leadership style assessments. There is a range available online. What sort of leader are you? Do you have any sense of how you express leadership in therapy? What is that like for you and where are the tensions? This may be material to explore in clinical supervision or even in some targeted personal therapy.

Your trauma history

If you find yourself having a strong response to the trauma content in a session with a client, try to take a longer break after that session, or whenever this is next possible. If a suitable colleague is present, you may also find it helpful to debrief, particularly if your strong emotional responses had some impact on your behaviour in the session. These responses to client material generally come unbidden and are no failing on our part. Noticing and reflecting on how they impact our work enables us to learn how to handle such responses with increasing skill.

To build your own awareness of your history and the sorts of stories that might produce strong responses for you, I recommend that you create your own trauma timeline. You could do this along the long edge of an A4 sheet of paper or a landscape document, or on a spreadsheet. Allocate a certain amount of space for each year of your life and then mark in any highly stressful events and anything involving actual or threatened death, injury, torture or sexual abuse, whether directed to you or to someone close to you. If you don't have much on the timeline, reflect back on any changes of house, school, and relationships, and any significant deaths of friends or family members. As you might expect, this can be a demanding exercise. If you think you need support to do this work, find yourself a therapist, even if only for a few sessions. Just like our clients, we have histories. These histories can affect our responses to our work. The better we know our histories and have digested that material, or are at least alert to its power, the better we can look after ourselves and manage this content in sessions. As with our longer-term thinking patterns, schemas, and defences, if you notice particular material regularly causing distress for you, you might consider some therapy of your own. We will return to these questions about our responses to trauma from another angle in Chapter 5, when we touch on vicarious trauma.

Attachment styles and personality traits

In each of these areas, and any other aspects of personality that seem relevant to your work as a therapist, a first step is a little self-education. If you don't know about your attachment styles, I recommend you complete an assessment. One such assessment is the Close Relationships Questionnaire on the Authentic Happiness website. If you know about your own attachment patterns, this can be an area for discussion with your clinical supervisor when the most recent work change is generating more stress for you than you might have anticipated.

If you haven't already explored your own personality structure, you might consider completing one of the free Big Five Personality dimensions tests or other reputable personality assessments online. Again, you might ask your clinical supervisor or colleagues for some brief support with an assessment and feedback.

Personal crises

If you find yourself struggling in the context of personal crises of one sort or another, remind yourself this is not a negative reflection on your work as a therapist. Remind yourself of previous personal crises that you have weathered successfully. As necessary, notice and challenge any negative self-talk, reflect on your needs, talk to your workplace and clinical supervisors, be diligent with your self-care, and attempt to negotiate changes to your work and family arrangements, so that you can continue to support your clients well and enjoy your work. There is also just the possibility that the combination of our personal circumstances and work may be too much to hold for a time. Sometimes, depending on the severity and duration of personal stressors and crises, we may need to take some leave, reduce hours, or even resign.

Managing physical and mental health

Whether or not you choose to disclose your health conditions to your workplace, if you want your career as a therapist to have longevity, I urge you to put in place your own self-management plan for any physical and mental health conditions that might affect your work as a therapist. This plan might include known triggers, early warning signs, action steps, and day-to-day maintenance tasks.

I have included on the next page a template for a self-management plan. I use this template with clients as a way of planning for relapse prevention for mental health conditions. You may wish to modify it to include physical health conditions as well. I use the last section of the plan myself. That question reads: *What are the maintenance, 'every day' or routine things you can do to care for yourself? What are the things you know help to keep your mood on an even keel? (Some examples might include, going to bed on time, eating well, talking to a friend, physical activity, relaxation exercises, or mindfulness practice.)* As I explain to clients when I introduce the plan to them, my plan includes getting regular exercise, sleeping well, and eating well. I tell them that when sometimes on a Friday afternoon I'm feeling particularly grumpy and having the thought that perhaps I shouldn't be a psychologist, I remember this plan. Usually that involves the rueful acknowledgement that there may have been some gaps in my self-care in that previous week: 'So there have been some days where I didn't get the exercise or sleep I planned, and where my food choices were less than ideal. OK,' I self-report my inner dialogue to my clients, 'so it's not a disaster. I just need to get back to doing the things I know I need to do'. As well as modelling a non-catastrophising, inner coach-leader to my clients, my aim is to model intentional planning for self-care. We know it is important for clients and it's important for us as therapists, as well. While any plan to manage physical and mental health issues will be limited, flawed, and in need of regular revision, an intentional plan says back to you and to colleagues who might be privy, that you take seriously the impact of the work on your person, and the impact of your person on the work.

- What are some of the events that might put you at risk of a relapse in terms of your mental health? (Some examples might include: bad news, family conflict or being reminded of a past event.)

- What are some of the warning signs that your mood is going downhill or that your levels of stress and anxiety are increasing? (You might list these in order, from the very first and smallest signs to the most obvious. You might even ask those who know you best what they notice.)

- When you notice these warning signs, what helps? What are some actions you can take to care for yourself? What strategies have you learnt or been reminded about that help? (You might list these in order, from the smallest things you know you need to do straightaway up to calling your psychologist/case manager/ general family medical practitioner /24-hour emergency numbers.)

- What are the maintenance, 'every day' or routine things you can do to care for yourself? What are the things you know help to keep your mood on an even keel? (Some examples might include, going to bed on time, eating well, talking to a friend, physical activity, relaxation exercises, or mindfulness practice.)

Workplace Tip

If you are in a position to influence decision-making in your workplace, encourage staff to care for their physical and mental health. Where this is possible, model this yourself, and work to provide avenues for physical and mental health care within the workplace.

Take-home message:

The better you understand the ways that your personal history, personality, and recent life experiences shape your attitudes and responses, the better you will be able to manage those responses when they arise in therapy. This is especially important if you suspect they are contributing to therapist distress or disenchantment. This level of understanding is an important foundation for managing your physical and mental health.

Where to next?

After two chapters focussed on the person of the therapist, we move to two chapters about the challenges of the work itself. We start with a chapter about situations when therapy work can be hard and slow.

Chapter 3

When the Work is Hard and Slow

In this exploration of the elements that contribute to therapist disenchantment, we have set the scene, looking at the aspects of our internal world and personal histories that provide resources for us but also tensions. Now, for a couple of chapters, we will consider some of the challenges of the work with clients themselves.

A fair proportion of the time, work with clients is hard, slow, or both hard and slow. In large part this is unavoidable and goes with the territory.

Sometimes the work is hard because you are hearing and holding hard things. One colleague I talked to about the idea of this book, challenged me: 'I've found a lot of such resources/training tend to oversimplify the pain and challenges that therapists experience in this space, prescribing yoga and mindfulness as a cure-all for what are complex political, spiritual and personal experiences of hardship shared.' She works with people who have experienced torture and trauma, many of whom have arrived as migrants and asylum seekers from war-torn countries.

While most of us will not work in such a challenging context, many of us will have some clients from such backgrounds. In addition, and not infrequently, our work involves journeying with people through deep and sensitive territory, including hurt, unfairness, and human unkindness. We may be sitting with clients who are wondering about meaning, purpose, and identity. They may be struggling with the possibility of forgiveness, regretting life choices, wrestling with small changes in seemingly intractable situations, or preparing for death. These conversations will affect us differently depending on where we are in our lives. If we have journeyed enough to recognise some of the territory, that may help us hear these questions rather than gloss over them. We don't need to be at the same stage as our clients, of course.

In fact, as we saw in 'Chapter 2: Know Yourself and Your History,' that may even be a risk at times. If clients are speaking into our own questions, this may be uncomfortable, and we may offer answers and distraction because we want to avoid the discomfort this brings. Even if these hard questions arise for the client primarily from a place of depression, they still need to be well acknowledged. In order to tolerate the discomfort and hold open a place for the client, we will need to draw deeply on our own resources for meaning and values. Although this work can be tremendously rewarding, it is not particularly well-paid and it is demanding. The person of the therapist is the medium. For this reason, among others, therapists need to take self-care seriously, and especially self-care at this deeper level of values and meaning. We will return to the challenge of deeper self-care in the last two chapters.

There are also many reasons why therapy work is slow. The first is that it takes time for the sort of trusting relationship to be established where people will share their more personal selves. A friend in pastoral ministry told me that it took at least two years working in a new congregation before some members shared at this level. As well, much of the time therapy is slow because normal healing takes time. Supporting people with grief is like this, whether it is a normal sort of grief or a more complicated one. This sort of work can't be rushed.

> *Philippa lost George after forty years of marriage. They married young and worked together in their small business. Philippa's adult self was shaped by life lived alongside George. He had been a kind man, but he now seemed perfect. She couldn't imagine life without him. Our work took time because it takes time to shape a new life. By contrast, Fred had been married to Lucy for around thirty years and had nursed her for the last five. He was convinced, though, that she had been having an affair in that last decade. He came to therapy grieving and angry. He had to talk it through outside his family. He came week after week, as he negotiated life without Lucy, communicated with his adult children, and sorted through her clothes and other possessions. Eventually, after a year, he and his family and close friends were*

> *able to have a ceremony remembering Lucy. They told stories, including the harder ones. Fred was able to lay Lucy to rest.*

While there are many reasons that therapy work can be hard or slow, the ones I have described above tend not to cause therapist disenchantment. In the main, this is because therapists can see that their work is making a positive difference. Reflecting back, I can think of at least five categories of work that are hard and slow and that are commonly experienced as stressful by therapists. By contrast to the client situations above, these clients often have longstanding mental health difficulties. As well, there is often a significant difference between the therapist's desire to be helpful and what is possible, not least because of limits to available funding or sessions. These situations include work with clients experiencing significant social disadvantage and multiple health issues, clients who behave 'badly,' those who are compelled to come to therapy, those who aren't yet ready to consider change, and clients with complicated presentations.

This is not an exhaustive list. You may well think of other types of work that belong here. Neither are these types of cases exclusive of one another. In fact, one of the reasons that a fair proportion of cases are hard and slow is that they have a lot going on. As you might expect, these cases are also made more complicated by what they trigger in us from our long-standing ways of being in the world and our histories. In addition, often the external context or constraints within which we work add to the challenge of work with these clients. In this chapter I provide a brief introduction to these cases, the ways they can affect us as therapists, and some suggestions. In all instances, though, it is particularly important to bring these cases to clinical supervision for support and to explore strategies.

Social disadvantage and multiple health issues

To begin with, there are the clients who attend while struggling with the effects of social disadvantage, or multiple health issues, or both. At the individual level, obtaining appropriate health care, employment, income, and housing can take time. It often takes much longer still for social injustice to be recognised and made right. These challenges can make it difficult for clients to focus on therapy. The slow pace of the work can then be dispiriting for client and therapist.

Suggestions

In practice, many of these clients fit into one of the four categories that follow. If this is the case, you might also refer to the strategies I outline there.

Although as therapists we have limited capacity to change these contexts for clients, it is appropriate for us to acknowledge them. Otherwise, we can end up further burdening our clients with the message that their health, or lack of it, is solely their responsibility. Yes, a degree of self-motivation and responsibility is always important in change, but there is a risk here of sliding into a very private and individual model of health and mental health that ignores the impact of community, culture, politics, and the environment.

With this broader context in mind, it may be that our client needs help with some sort of injustice or systemic discrimination. Our validation and solidarity may be essential in their healing process. Some clients will need you to advocate for them. In an Australian context, this most commonly involves supporting clients while they go through a work injury insurance claim process. This experience of adversarial legal processes can be very much like that represented in Charles Dickens's *Bleak House*, absorbing time, focus, hope, morale, and money. Nonetheless, clients who make it through with a successful outcome often feel at least temporarily better, both to be without the struggle but also to have acknowledgement of their claim and some measure of justice.

This observation, that a successful outcome in an application for workplace compensation can improve the mental health of a client, invites us to reflect on the criteria we use to define health, how we think it is achieved, and how we measure success. As well, on all those occasions where we are focussing largely on a person's thoughts or feelings in the moment, rather than on their larger context, we are probably missing out on places where positive change might be possible, or is occurring.

The classic medical model of health sees health as an absence of disease or diagnosis and relies heavily on medical science. Psychiatrists, psychologists, and clinically trained mental health workers are often drawn into this model by training that focuses on evidence-based interventions. The message we receive from the medical model of health is that, if we apply the treatment as intended, and clients follow it appropriately, a certain percentage of clients will get better, at least temporarily. Now, there is much to be said for the knowledge we have in this area, and for the effectiveness of our treatments. One of the serious limitations to the model, however, is that not all clients can use our therapies, or use them as intended, and not all benefit. In addition, many clients will benefit to some extent but remain with mental health symptoms, or benefit temporarily and then relapse. Often this occurs where a client's personal history or current life circumstances are so complicated that it is hardly surprising and in fact deeply misleading to suggest that sessions with a therapist, however empathic, skilful or evidence-based, could entirely shift symptoms.

As part of our original training, most of us will also have encountered the bio-psycho-social model, and its extension, the bio-psycho-socio-spiritual model. As therapists we know full well that the whole context of a person's life affects their mental health. Usually, though, our training did not encourage us to see this insight as a basis for planning therapy and mental health interventions and for assessing outcomes. If from busyness, habit, or reporting requirements, we only use quantitative measures of mental health symptoms, we will miss changes that happen in other parts of a client's life. Perhaps they are exercising a little more or have re-engaged with a hobby? Perhaps they are more in contact with their family or a social network or their faith community than they were? Perhaps they have found work? It is possible that in these circumstances their quantitative measures of mood may improve as well. There is good reason why exercise, engaging with valued activities, and re-engaging with social networks are so consistently effective in improving mood. However, even if quantitative symptom measures don't change much in the course of therapy, that doesn't mean that it has been ineffective in addressing the bio-psycho-social dimensions of clients' lives. Changes in exercise, activities, social networks or vocational status often affect how a person thinks about themselves and their ability to cope, and how they understand their history.

Another model that can be helpful here is the social model of health, which examines all the elements that contribute to health, including social, cultural, political, and environmental factors. One community health centre I worked at proactively espoused this perspective when staff planned services. This contributed to the development of a community choir, classes about accessing nutritional food, and a referral network to support clients needing employment, accommodation, and advocacy. There is much overlap between this model and that of the bio-psycho-socio-spiritual model, but it has the added benefit of considering a wider range of factors that bear on the lives and wellbeing of our clients.

All the connections in a person's life—including to family, neighbours, and community—impact on their physical and mental health. Sometimes—and perhaps often—the most effective ways to get change when therapy work is hard and slow involve widening the habitually narrow lens of the therapist to this broader realm of connections. If a relationship can change, a client's mood might improve, even if life is very tough in many respects. If they find a job, their debt-related stress may drop a little and their self-confidence may increase. If their nutrition and food security is improved, this may similarly make a difference to their health and mood. If they have somewhere to spend time with people, where they are valued, be this at a men's group, like a Men's Shed, or choir, this may similarly make a positive difference to how they feel about themselves and their lives.

I'm thinking of a client, Fernanda. In the four years we worked together, she slowly absorbed some ideas about how to manage her mood and anxiety. Except for brief periods of respite, she continued to report a high level of anxiety and low mood symptoms and near weekly thoughts of suicide. She found interaction with other people difficult and was frequently simmering with rage at perceived slights and threats from others. If I considered her situation based on symptoms alone, both of us could have felt discouraged. If I stepped back for a moment and considered our work and her progress by these two other models, a different picture emerged. In those four years, Fernanda eventually found a psychiatrist she trusted. She didn't always follow his advice, but she turned up to see him regularly. She had a lot of worry about her health, and dealt with numerous actual and feared conditions. At the end of those four years, however, all her health conditions were well treated and stable. Despite all her inquiries and tests, nothing serious was identified and she was beginning to believe that at least some of her symptoms might be related to anxiety. Even more significantly, during these years she re-established contact with two family members, both of whom displayed considerable understanding about her difficulties attending family events. As well, despite much anxiety and frustration along the way, she wrestled with government agencies about her income and accommodation, and both were now secure. None of these things were the case when she first came to see me. Viewed from this perspective, she made substantial progress.

This brings us to the idea of social prescribing. Originating from Dr Sam Everington's East London clinic, the Bromley-by-Bow Centre, it started as an experiment to see if patients who were prescribed some sort of social activity did any better than clients prescribed medication alone. It is hard, of course, to research this sort of treatment in a randomised placebo-controlled double-blind way. That said, people report gains—this makes sense—and for patients with very complicated lives and where resources for treatment are limited, this approach also has the benefit of encouraging the health of a civil society that can be very much under threat. If this brief description of social prescribing appeals to you, I recommend that you read the chapter about it in Johann Hari's book, *Lost Connections: Uncovering the real causes of depression—and the unexpected solutions* (2018), and that you investigate social prescribing projects in your area.

Clients behaving 'badly'

I'm guessing that many therapists will have seen this title and flicked straight to this section. Perhaps this is a shadow place for therapists. We care about clients, but at times we are also frustrated and frightened by them. These are usually our most unwell clients; the ones who have experienced the most significant trauma. We know that a lot of their testing behaviours come out of their places of hurt and often from barely understood childhood patterns, but it's still hard not to call it 'bad' behaviour—it *feels* bad—and the line between behaviour we might rightly label to clients as completely understandable and even heroic in its place, and that which is also maladaptive and destructive, is very fine indeed. As therapists, we walk that line with clients, being gentle and respectful, but also consistently eliciting the downsides of such behaviours and working with their motivation to do differently, to disarm just a little, and to add some other behavioural options to their repertoire.

Not turning up

One of the most common categories of 'bad' behaviour is that of turning up late or not turning up or giving late notice. This is often extremely frustrating and demoralising for therapists, especially when their income depends on clients turning up, and when other clients could have attended in their place. This is in a related category to turning up unannounced with paperwork to complete or asking for a letter at short notice. Both often come from the chronic problems with concentration, memory, and organisation that can accompany anxiety and depression. Both often also arise from patterns of avoiding discomfort. To make matters more complicated for therapists, these are often unconscious patterns in our clients, a form of implicit memory in the shape of resistance. This sort of passive-aggressive avoidance may have been one of the few ways they could protect themselves from aversive experiences as a child. Unfortunately, it is likely to be causing problems for them in various aspects of their adult lives.

Suggestions

I have a colleague who takes the time to text or call all clients the day before their sessions, commenting that levels of anxiety and low mood make it hard to be organised. Speaking out of my high standards and love of order, I tend to argue back to him that if people can't manage to attend, they need encouragement to work on that skill. After all, no one makes excuses for someone who doesn't turn up to the hotel room they have booked. I grant you, of course, that turning up to a holiday may feel quite different from turning up to see your therapist, who you know will ask you again about the uncomfortable and even painful places in your life. Each therapist develops their own practices for working with clients about such boundary violations. As these patterns in clients not infrequently intersect with difficulties in assertiveness and patterns of self-sacrifice in therapists, patterns that can easily flip the therapists from victim to perpetrator, feeling put-upon to behaving punitively, I recommend that you proactively develop a clear and documented process that avoids the extremes of indulgence and punitiveness. The automatic text message with a reminder of appointment details and prompt to reply YES or NO seems almost ubiquitous now. From experience though, a consistent percentage of clients do not reply, or claim they have replied when no reply message has been received. A high proportion send a NO at short notice and a smaller proportion send one in the moments before the appointment. In combination with the automated text message or as a standalone approach in low technology settings, I have found that being very clear at the beginning of therapy, verbally and in writing, then having a one-off grace occasion for every client, where I speak to them myself about the consequences, very much reduces subsequent 'misbehaviour'. That said, the one centre where we advertised that any non-attendance after the first occasion would produce a bill for the entire fee, almost immediately eliminated this behaviour. Perhaps hotels know what they are doing when they take a deposit and our credit card details.

Anger

Another category of 'bad' behaviour is when clients take out their anger on therapists. Sometimes the therapist has made a mistake or misjudgement. Sometimes the therapist's behaviour was unremarkable but was perceived as hurtful or neglectful, perhaps in a context where it reminded the client of trauma. Often the client is angry for other reasons. Sometimes the truth is a combination. Sometimes the anger is partly hidden or hinted at in small passive-aggressive behaviours—like being late. More often, it is there overtly in the room, on a spectrum from owned and discussable to entirely blaming and undiscussable. One client sat for almost the entire session in silent fury with me that our available government-funded sessions were coming to an end. A colleague wrote:

Early in my work in private practice I had a first session with a female client in her thirties. As was the way with this centre, I had about three minutes to look at the referral before we met. If I had absorbed it carefully, I might have better understood the implications. It mentioned that she had a traumatic brain injury (TBI), alcohol use disorder and a history of being violently verbally abusive to therapists. I noticed the TBI, alcohol and anger but in passing. In our opening conversation my client was very slurred in speech—something that was not present at our second session. I was conscious that she might be alcohol-affected and that it might be best to defer our conversation to a later date. Stumblingly, acknowledging I knew very little about her situation, I said I was struggling to follow what she was saying. I saw a number of things on her referral that might be contributing to communication difficulties, including her head injury but also possibly alcohol use. If it was alcohol use, perhaps it might be better to reschedule. As you can imagine, it is very hard to get that sort of question right, even in the best of circumstances. What followed was a tirade of abuse, blame, attack, and belittling. She was very good at what she did and I was left winded and shaken by the verbal onslaught. She was not physically violent, but this could easily have been a risk, especially with a new and unknown client.

Anger is tricky to deal with because of the strong energy it generates both for the client and therapist, and the increased likelihood that a rush of blood to the head for one or other will result in words or actions we regret in a calmer moment.

Suggestions

This is certainly a situation where therapists need to practice all the skills they can muster—empathy, validation, but also centeredness and clear-sightedness, along with basic anger management for both parties. In situations where I have been in error or can see how my behaviour might have been misconstrued, I have found Marsha Linehan's guidelines helpful: in essence, our role is to model a healthy way of managing anger. Knowing how exquisitely we as humans are tuned to the emotions of others, these guidelines encourage us to pay particular attention to our own facial expression, body language and tone. Working as best we can to convey openness, calm and caring, we will hear out the client, where they are able to communicate without verbal abuse, and then express genuine understanding and validation for the response. Then we may acknowledge our role clearly, and with an appropriate apology, or briefly explain any misunderstanding while expressing regret for the distress that resulted. My experience has been that in most instances this is very effective.

For situations where a client is being abusive and out of control, the three warnings method seems to work. I learnt this from Lifeline. On these telephone lines, counsellors can be on the receiving end of verbal abuse from callers, the anonymity of the call giving some clients licence to be abusive to caring strangers. At Lifeline, staff were advised that if verbal abuse was directed at a counsellor, he should immediately, respectfully, but clearly, state that while it is normal to be angry, abusive language directed to counsellors was unacceptable and if it continued, he would end the call. Some clients would pull back at that stage. At the second instance, the therapist would advise that if it happened again, he would end the call. Then, if there was a third instance, the therapist would end the call immediately. Most adults don't like being told what to do, and this is even more so for angry people who have already veered into abusive language. So, any intervention in this area is unlikely to end well. What it may do, at very least, is limit how much abuse a counsellor receives. It is also just possible that it underlines for the caller and counsellor a basic rule of civil human behaviour: that verbal abuse is unacceptable.

Considering the earlier story of the client with a TBI, I recommend that you read all referrals as carefully as your time permits, and consider what safety plans you need to put in place.

Each therapist will develop their own practices for safety. Consider sitting out of the way of the door, so clients can readily leave. As well, be prepared to leave the room yourself, in an announced and boundary-setting way, or citing the need to collect some paperwork, depending on the degree to which the situation feels physically safe. In centres where they do not have duress alarms, consider having your own alarm device present and accessible. I have never needed to use mine, but there have been situations with new clients where I have been grateful to know it was there. If you can, arrange to never be alone in your centre with new clients and with male clients with whom you feel ill at ease. I have experienced some pressure from centres that were keen to accommodate clients, especially at the margins of the day when centres were otherwise unstaffed, but I understand that pressure to reflect a want of imagination and a neglect of occupational health and safety by those workplaces. Just occasionally, clients assault or kill therapists. It's rare, of course, and I do not want therapists reading this to live and practice with that possibility at the centre of their awareness. Instead, I'm advocating that we put processes in place that acknowledge and address the possibility, so that we can get on with and continue our work in safety.

Self-harm and suicidal behaviours

The third category of 'bad' behaviour, if you can call it that, are the clients who self-harm, or who engage in para-suicidal or frankly suicidal behaviours. I know that it is controversial to call this 'bad' behaviour, as it almost always arises from considerable distress. As noted earlier, this is complicated for therapists because these are often our most unwell clients, and this behaviour is not uncommon in the stabilisation phase of trauma work. I am using the word 'bad' here to signify how intensely stressful such behaviours are for therapists—and, of course, for the other people in a client's life. We are wired as humans such that behaviours that are life-threatening or that we perceive as life-threatening, generate a very strong anxiety response. That is supposed to happen, so that—ideally—the person who is at risk can be made safe again. A strong anxiety response is hard enough on the therapist when it happens once, but it is harder still when a client has a chronic pattern of para-suicidal, or frankly suicidal, behaviours. These are some of the hardest situations with which therapists have to work.

Suggestions

I suggest that you do not carry these clients alone. Make sure you have adequate support and supervision. If you don't have that support, do whatever you can to stop seeing these clients until you have the support you need.

If you work for an organisation, do what you can to be familiar with its policies for working with clients who report thoughts of suicide or self-harm.

Have a plan in place about how you will ask about risk and respond to reports of recent self-harm or suicidality or future plans. Talk this through with your clinical supervisor and commit it to memory.

With this plan in mind, have tools available for assessing risk, planning with clients how to keep safe, and calling emergency services if needed.

With every new client, before they tell their story, talk about the limits of confidentiality associated with your service, including if you are concerned about their safety, or that of someone else. Document that you have had that conversation with them. I say, 'This service is confidential. There are some limits. They include: … If I'm concerned about your safety or someone else's, I may need to talk to someone else about that, but if it is possible, I'll try to talk to you about my concerns.' I use this wording, because it usually puts people at their ease to know I'll try to talk to them about my concerns. It also gives me permission to breach their confidentially, without telling them, if I really need to do so. In my years of practice, I have found that most of the time when I need to reach out for additional supports, clients give their agreement. In a busy private practice, this could happen as often as every couple of months. I have only ever needed to breach the confidentiality of a small percentage of clients, but this still happened around once a year. In both instances, the small effort involved in having upfront conversations about confidentiality is worth it. Keep in mind that, depending on the country you work in, somewhere between 10 and 20 percent of the population have thoughts of suicide in any given year, and this number will be higher among therapy clients. I have learnt that having in place a structure and understanding with all clients that I return to if needed, saves a whole lot of stress in situations where a client does later report self-harm or thoughts of suicide. It also creates an opportunity to provide psychoeducation to clients about suicide. I have observed that this means the ice is already broken, as it were, and that it is easier for them to come back to me about this topic than if it had never been broached.

Whenever needed, and ideally with every new client who reports depression, ask about self-harm and suicide, provide some psychoeducation about how these behaviours and thoughts can be more present when someone is depressed, and be ready to assess risk and tailor a response to the need. Document any risk assessment you conduct and any plan you create with the client. Consult with a colleague or an emergency service if needed. Document the outcome of that conversation. Follow-up with the client at a pre-agreed time. As needed, repeat the assessment, planning, consultation, documentation, and follow-up.

As soon as you can, and from time to time in your career, do professional development reading or courses on how to respond to self-harm and suicide. As this area generates considerable stress for therapists, the more skilled you are, the better this will be for you and your career.

The compelled, the complainers, and the clients

Somewhere in my training a lecturer told our class that people who attend therapy are either compelled, complainers, or clients. By 'compelled,' he meant those many people who come to therapy primarily because they have been sent by others; by 'complainers,', he meant people who spend most of the session complaining about other people or circumstances; and by 'clients' he meant people who arrive at therapy ready to work on their issues and make change. The first two groups can be particularly challenging for therapists, and they are surprisingly common. We only wish that more people arrived as 'clients.'

The compelled

The most extreme versions of the compelled, I imagine, are those who are sent to therapy in prison. Colleagues tell me, however, that with fewer distractions in their lives, prisoners are often more motivated to talk to a therapist or to work on their issues. One step down from there might be the people in the community who have been told that they need to attend therapy as part of a community corrections order. They are not actually obliged to turn up but there will be significant negative consequences if they don't. That work can be complicated, because sometimes the client has very serious offending behaviours, including abuse and violence, and they may not see any need to change those behaviours. Oftentimes, that work is also complicated for therapists by the expectations of the law enforcement or corrections staff who want the client to turn up and to be treated for the behaviours of concern. In a private treatment context though, a therapist cannot compel attendance and has different imperatives from corrections staff. They can work with a client to build their motivation, but if a client doesn't attend or engage, that is the client's choice. Fortunately, for most therapists, our compelled clients come in other forms. These are the many people sent by parents, children, friends, partners, and colleagues. Usually, they announce that they have been 'sent' early in the work, and they have a very different view of their situation from that of the person who sent them. Almost universally they do not think they have the problem 'diagnosed' by their loved ones, and as such, they come prepared to defend themselves in the therapy space.

Suggestions

John, a wonderful counsellor trainer I met in the fourth year of my psychology training, shared with us the importance of first acknowledging with the client whatever compulsion was there for them to attend, and then conveying your genuine desire for the therapy space to be useful for them. Other people in their lives might have agendas for them, of course, but what does the client think about these goals? What matters to them? Could those things instead be the focus of some work together? I have found that in most instances this approach will successfully engage the otherwise reluctant client. Sometimes, then, we eventually return to the issues that resulted in them being 'sent' to therapy in the first place.

The complainers

Then there are the complainers. These clients tend to experience a lot of distress in their relationships with others but, for various reasons, they do not think they have any responsibility for that conflict or any power to change it. In my experience, many clients in this category will naturally move to the point of being open to taking some action if they have had an opportunity to be well heard. That said, in the context of limited sessions and subsidised work, about once a year I have a conversation with a client and send a letter to their referring general family medical practitioner noting that the continuing content of sessions is complaint, that the sessions do not seem to be helping, and that if anything, sessions are making the client's sense of grievance worse. I usually write that while I'm willing to continue to provide supportive counselling rather than structured therapy, my hope would be to encourage the client to engage in the enterprise of change.

Suggestions

Perhaps the most powerful tools I've encountered for assessing a client's openness to change are Stephen Covey's circles of concern and influence. This diagram has two concentric circles—that is, a small circle inside a larger circle. The larger circle represents the many things about which we are concerned and the small circle, the subset of those issues over which we have influence. In discussing Habit 1: Be Proactive, in *The 7 Habits of Highly Effective People*, Covey recommends that proactive people focus intently on the things over which they have influence, and that over time they make their circle of influence grow by gradually considering more skilful ways of addressing issues in their circle of concern. As well as a self-management tool, this is also one of the most powerful stress management tools in my armoury. John, the counsellor-trainer I mentioned earlier, suggested asking clients to write down in the respective circles the things that cause them stress over which they have no influence or control—the circle of concern—and then things that cause them stress over which they have some influence or control—the circle of influence. Once this was complete, he suggested asking clients how they felt when they considered both sets of stress, starting with the outer circle, that is, the one over which they have no control or influence. Generally, people feel far worse about the issues in the outer circle. Sometimes people feel stressed about the issues in the inner circle because they know that they require action and they feel dispirited. Mostly though, people feel far less stressed and even empowered when they focus on what is under their control or influence. If this is what your client tells you, that is a sign that you might have a customer or client on your hands and not a complainer.

Now in my experience, most clients come as an admixture of two or more of these categories and need a little work to increase their motivation for change. Change is hard: much harder than most of us realise or are prepared to admit. Nonetheless, as Henry David Thoreau writes, it is a miracle that is taking place in every instant. If a client comes with some openness, that can usually be nurtured in therapy. In my work for Quit Victoria, the section of the Cancer

Council Victoria providing telephone counselling to people contemplating changes to smoking behaviours, we routinely used Motivational Interviewing. This is a gem of a therapy for supporting someone to make change, especially change to longstanding behaviours. It works to increase a person's own sense of motivation and to reduce their resistance to change, while getting them to think more about the possibility of change. If you are looking for additional skills for working with motivation, I can recommend Motivational Interviewing to you. There are frequently short courses available and the original text, *Motivational Interviewing: Preparing People to Change Addictive Behavior* (1991), by William Miller and Stephen Rollnick is very accessible.

Complex cases

Clients who feel 'stuck'

Really complex cases come in many and varied forms. For our purposes, I will distinguish between two types of clients. Both have experienced one or more significant traumas and their experience of emotional struggle continues pretty much unabated. The first group have at least some early experiences of emotional resilience and some solid family or community supports. They only rarely have or act on thoughts of suicide, but their quality of life is poor. It is as though they, and we, are stuck. Some contributors here can be:

- melancholic or endogenous depression, or a client who is deeply identified with an interpersonal hurt or their diagnosis and has little sense of an identity beyond it;
- clients with such intense anxiety that they process material from sessions very slowly, and so need to return again and again to be reminded of and to practice skills; and
- clients dealing with some level of cognitive challenge, either congenital or acquired, that subtly or more dramatically affects their ability to take in information and to apply it.

Suggestions

There is considerable overlap among the presentations that contribute to therapeutic work being hard and slow. Sometimes, for example, someone with very entrenched depression is also primarily a complainer. If you have a client who is 'stuck' and who also has elements of other categories, consider the strategies already mentioned above.

Remind yourself of clients with similar backgrounds with whom you have worked successfully. In fact, I encourage you to collect cards, notes, or comments of appreciation from clients. Generally, therapists do not receive exuberant expressions of thanks from clients. Most of the time, the rewards and gifts of therapy come in seeing improvement. When evidence of improvement is hard to come by, it is good to remind ourselves of past successes and past words of appreciation.

Sometimes, you will need to acknowledge to yourself that this is and would be challenging work, regardless of your skill and experience. Assure yourself you are doing the best you can and that it is unlikely any of your colleagues would be doing any better in that situation. Perhaps what is in your control is the possibility of changing your perspective. We will return to this in Chapter 7.

Carefully review, revise, and follow your formulation, that is, your understanding of what is going on for this client and as a result, what therapy approaches make sense.

Ask yourself what resources your therapy of choice has for thinking about someone being stuck. It is very tempting when a feeling of 'stuckness' continues in therapy to make negative moral judgements about the client or about yourself. One great benefit to Schema Therapy, Internal Family Systems Therapy, and other therapies including Gestalt Therapy, which consider parts or elements of a person, is the way they allow us—the client and ourselves—to see that *a particular part of the client is stuck*. This isn't all of them by any means, or they wouldn't be coming to therapy in the first place. Once we and they are able to distinguish that part from the client themselves, other insights flow and an unexpected energy is often released as well. If your primary therapy doesn't include resources for this work, you might find helpful Scott Kellogg's work, *Transformational Chairwork: Using psychotherapeutic dialogues in clinical practice* (2015).

If you haven't already done so, talk to your clinical supervisor about the case. If you need to, have a second or third conversation.

Consider requesting a medication review by the client's general family medical practitioner or even by a psychiatrist.

Consider a change of therapy. For example, sometimes the person has received as much improvement from CBT as they can. They might benefit from a move to Schema Therapy or some other therapy that would help them understand and contemplate change to longstanding patterns. It can be helpful to have several therapies up your sleeve, as it were.

If you don't use the sort of therapy that might be relevant, you might learn it. For example, clients who have experienced sexual assault may be unable to use Exposure Therapy. They may need Cognitive Processing Therapy (CPT). On the other hand, CPT requires literacy, a willingness to do daily written tasks, and a settled enough life to make this possible. Eye-Movement Desensitisation and Reprocessing (EMDR) might be needed in cases where these preconditions are not present.

It takes time and expense to learn and practice new therapies. If the client in front of you needs skills you don't have, and they are willing to transfer, make an appropriate and professional referral to someone who does. It is important for your wellbeing and that of the client to work within the limits of your competence.

If, for this or other reasons, the client is a bad match with you at this point, neither of you have failed. As Louis Cozolino writes, perhaps you are preparing a client for therapeutic success with another therapist.

Clients presenting in repeated crisis

The second type of complex case is marked by the client presenting to most sessions in crisis, or reporting a recent crisis. These crises may include self-harm, para-suicidal behaviours or frankly suicidal behaviours. With these clients, it feels nearly impossible to come up with a plan, because there are so many diagnoses, the target and presenting issues seems to change every session, and the client is often so distressed that a significant portion of the session is taken up with crisis management. The vast majority of clients who present in these ways have a complex form of trauma: they experienced highly stressful events in their childhood, sometimes including life-threatening events, and then in their teens, twenties, and later adult lives they have experienced further layers of trauma. The interactions of daily life trigger intense and prolonged distress that then cause them to behave in ways that complicate things further. Many have Post-traumatic Stress Disorder and many have either traits of one or more personality disorders, or they meet some or all criteria for Borderline Personality Disorder or Emotionally Unstable Personality Disorder. In all instances, it is hard to obtain appropriate and sufficient therapy. Services may not exist in the government sector, or waiting lists may be very long. The quickest way to access treatment may be through private health insurance, which is often prohibitively expensive. This means that many of our clients never get the full dose of treatment they would need. Instead, we are doing the best we can with limited resources. This is hard work for both the client and the therapist.

Suggestions

As with all the other client types described in this chapter, see your clinical supervisor regularly about these clients.

Talk with your client candidly and collaboratively about the evidence-base for treatments and the limits of what you can offer given the time and resources available. Engage them with planning and thinking about what you do in therapy and how to make it relevant to them. This is an important part of establishing informed consent for treatment and being clear about expectations. Consider using brief elements of Dialectical Behaviour Therapy (DBT) or Schema Therapy, even if this is less than ideal. Perhaps a change to a time-limited therapy like Cognitive Analytic Therapy (CAT) might be helpful. Sometimes, after such conversations, clients go elsewhere for treatment, say for a specific condition or therapy. At other times, you may need to wait until a new funding year, when you have more sessions available. At other times still, perhaps after some years, clients may find sufficient income or support to afford the insurance so they can attend more sessions with you or a specialist service.

It was this group of clients Marsha Linehan had in mind when she developed DBT. She recognised clients were routinely presenting in crisis and that clients and therapists found it almost impossible to make progress. To address these challenges, Linehan developed a therapy where clients attend weekly group skill-building sessions and fortnightly individual therapy. Over the course of four terms, the skill-based groups focus on learning crisis management or distress tolerance, emotional regulation, mindfulness, and interpersonal effectiveness skills, as well as how to apply these instead of potentially harmful behaviours. The individual therapy is intended to help the person apply the skills they have learnt to the crisis that occurred in the last fortnight. Having seen this therapy delivered by a dedicated team myself, Linehan's treatment model is compelling. Some people need to attend for two years. Others still need some sort of graduate program helping them to address trauma specifically, once they have the skills to tolerate it, and beyond that, to structure what DBT calls 'a life worth living'.

Similarly, when clients present as more stable but with debilitating long-term interpersonal patterns, weekly to fortnight Schema Therapy, Mentalisation-Based Therapy, or other longer-term psychotherapies may help.

Workplace Tip

If you are in a position to influence decision-making in your workplace, do what you can to ensure your organisation has clear and useable processes for assessing, documenting, and responding to suicidal ideation and self-harm. Be particularly mindful of workers who are working with such clients and do what you can to provide support for them so that they are not carrying this weight alone.

Take-home message:

When therapy work is hard and slow in these ways, pause, remember your successes, reflect on what you are doing, see your clinical supervisor, develop a plan, try it out, review it, and repeat this process as necessary. Try to be as kind to yourself and your client as you can be.

Where to next?

The next chapter considers three aspects of therapy work that commonly contribute to therapist stress.

CHAPTER 4

Transference and Countertransference, Vicarious Trauma, and Moral Injury

A couple of years ago a client started coming for sessions, although often with big gaps in between. She wanted my help with some government processes but completely rejected any of the options I offered her. In most sessions during that first year, I felt a strong urge to run from the room and leave the profession for good. The first time very much caught me by surprise, but when it happened again, I became curious. I've since come to understand that I was experiencing a very strong countertransference response. It was only as I came to know her story that I realised that she was transferring onto me her former abusive partner, who had constantly set about to humiliate her. She was transferring this on to me because, unknown to me, the things I was asking her to do reminded her of her partner. Specifically, to her I felt—and was—in a position of power that made her feel very vulnerable. When I understood this, I realised that her very defensive response made me feel like I was harming her and being a bad therapist. My response to that feeling was near catastrophic. If I was doing harm then all I wanted to do was leave the work and never darken the doors of the place again. What strikes me in retrospect was how all of this was unconscious and how intense the response was. It took all my concentration to stay in the room and to behave professionally and it took over a year before I understood what was going on. I had to tolerate the strong responses, knowing that they contained important information, and not necessarily the information that I needed to leave my work.

In this chapter, in particular, we touch on three of the more severe and direct ways in which the work affects therapists: transference and countertransference, illustrated in the story above from one therapist, vicarious trauma, and moral injury. There are small libraries of books and journal articles on each of these processes and how to treat them. I include here a brief introduction and some pointers.

Transference and countertransference

Transference refers to any distortion in therapy that occurs because of the client's unconscious. This includes but is not limited to the things that a client projects or transfers onto a therapist, often some attitude or role held by a significant care-giver. Similarly, countertransference refers to any distortion in therapy that occurs because of the therapist's unconscious. This includes but goes far beyond the unconscious responses the therapist has to transference from the client. By this second definition, you will see that much of what we discussed in the first two chapters, on our thinking patterns and personal history, could be material for countertransference, especially if we have no regular way of reflecting on our responses to what happens in sessions.

Perhaps the most familiar pattern for me is one where a client transfers onto me a caregiving role and then behaves in a somewhat demanding and helpless way, insisting that I help them. I have noticed that my automatic response is to think that the person is being needy when I think they are quite capable. Before I was alert to this pattern, I would often respond saying something like, 'I think you already know a lot about how to handle this situation'. Rather than prompting the client to draw on his own resourcefulness, this sort of response often produced still more helpless and demanding behaviours in the client, along with a dash of defensiveness. It has taken me years to recognise and understand this pattern so that I can restrain myself and respond more flexibly and skilfully. Sometimes that sees me begin with noticing the client's emotions, reflecting them back as appropriate: 'It seems like you are feeling a bit overwhelmed with all the things you are juggling at present?' Sometimes I follow that up with, 'What's the part of X that's concerning you most right now?', or an appropriate variant. Usually that opens a way forward.

Far more than most therapists realise, transference and countertransference affect how we interact with clients and how we feel about our work. These processes tend to be most common and powerful when we are working with clients who have experienced trauma, especially developmental or ongoing traumas. These patterns regularly interfere with the work, whether expressed by clients around attendance, fees, their seeming expectations of therapists, or projections onto therapist. When these patterns are not recognised as transference, it is hard for therapists to help a clients get their needs met by other means. Countertransference also interferes with therapy when unwittingly therapists find themselves responding more like the client's former antagonist or abuser—angry, frustrated, dismissive—than the helper we would like to be. As well, as Hawkins and Shohet write, when a therapist does not own their own motivations and needs, it is hard to address them in other ways, without using clients to make us feel good about ourselves, or making clients carry around bits of ourselves, such as our projections of absent but important others.

Suggestions

As noted, both processes—transference and countertransference—are largely unconscious and as a result, often need considerable reflection to recognise and understand. As these responses happen in most sessions and throughout sessions, it pays to be alert to them and ready to ask yourself the question, 'What did I notice?' It is worth noticing any changes in emotional tone, places of frustration, and responses that feel familiar. If you are someone who keeps a reflection journal, a professional version would be a good place for these reflections. If you make notes in advance of your clinical supervision sessions, that can also be a good place to record your observations. Ideally, develop a practice of writing about this material as soon after a session as possible.

If you are noticing difficulties in the work with a client but are struggling to put your finger on them, revisit your case conceptualisation or formulation and consider the place of resistance and other defences in the client's response.

Consider the impression that the client is likely to make on others, and is likely to have made on you already, even if you haven't expressed this to yourself. As well, consider the impression that you are likely to make on others and the largely unconscious attitudes that clients may form toward you. Given what you know about your client's history, are there people in their life of whom you might remind them? Similarly, does the client remind you of anyone in your life, even a former and memorable client, if only through their life stage or presenting issue? I'm thinking, for example, of the number of mature female counsellors at a counselling agency who reported what they recognised as maternal feelings of care and frustration toward the young adults presenting at their service. These forms of association often find expression in transference and countertransference.

The more we are alert for these patterns and know our most familiar responses, the better we will be able to manage these in sessions and attend to self-care afterwards.

If this area of transference and countertransference is unfamiliar to you and of interest, please consider exploring it further. One place to start might be Louis Cozolino's *The Making of a Therapist: A practical guide for the inner journey*. Cozolino offers many insights for early-career therapists and reflects extensively on transference, countertransference, and working with client defences and resistance patterns.

Workplace Tip

If you are in a position to influence decision-making in your workplace, do what you can to encourage quality professional development training that acknowledges the three areas in this chapter, transference and countertransference, vicarious trauma, and moral injury.

Vicarious trauma

The current working definitions of Post-traumatic Stress Disorder (PTSD) relate specifically to people who have experienced actual or threatened death, serious injury, or sexual violence. Alternatively, a person may have witnessed such a traumatic event occur to someone else, or they may have learnt about such an experience by someone close to them. Finally, they may have been repeatedly exposed to the adverse details of such traumatic events as part of their work. Common examples include first responders to accidents or police who are repeatedly exposed to the details of child abuse. Whether or not someone is given a diagnosis after such an experience relates to the level of re-experiencing, avoidance, and hyper-vigilance symptoms, and the level of cognitive and emotional symptoms they experience related to the event, one month later and beyond.

While the definition itself includes the possibility that learning about an experience can cause PTSD, generally therapists are not 'close to' clients in the way where their own responses would meet this definition. Some exceptions to this may happen in instances where a trauma occurs to a client during our work with them, when we have a pre-existing and caring relationship to them. In addition, particularly at times of man-made or natural disaster, therapists may be working in their own communities providing psychological first aid, and are either exposed to life threatening circumstances themselves, and/or repeatedly exposed to the adverse experiences of others. Many therapists had experiences like this while they worked during COVID-19 lockdowns.

It is important to add here that the terms 'traumatic stress' and 'post-traumatic stress' capture a range of significant stressors that are much wider than those included in a diagnosis of PTSD. For example, some forms of workplace bullying or harassment and family conflict, while not events indicated in the diagnosis of PTSD, are most definitely experienced as traumatic by clients, who often have similar symptoms to clients with a diagnosis of PTSD. As well, exposure to the trauma story of another can have a traumatising effect on the hearer. Vicarious trauma is the term generally used for this experience, and also for the accumulated effects of hearing many trauma stories, the common experience of therapists. Depending on the volume and severity of stories and the amount of content related to actual or threatened death, serious injury or sexual violence, this may produce symptoms that meet criteria for PTSD. Much of the time, though, these responses are similar to those present in PTSD but of less duration or intensity than that needed for a diagnosis.

Our vulnerability to vicarious trauma, whether we are therapists or private citizens, is associated with what in other respects is a very important part of our ability to survive: our capacity to interpret and identify with the responses of others, and especially to read their facial expression and vocal tone. We are acutely sensitive to such cues. When life was more primitive, this will have been important for safety. If you have ever watched meercats in the zoo, you can see it in operation. If one individual detects a risk and conveys distress, others seeing this catch something of the distress themselves, and act to keep themselves safe. This sensitivity to and absorption of emotional states happens all the time and in less high-stakes situations as well, and seems to be wired into us. Being calm, smiling at a baby, and speaking to her in soothing tones, helps her to settle. As she settles, we feel calmer as well. We co-regulate our emotions. Lovers do this too, when agitated, aroused, or simply holding each other. This capacity is also a tremendous tool in therapy. It helps us empathise with words and gestures, as we listen to words but also for emotional cues. This capacity helps us to soothe clients, as we use our own calm tone, facial expression, and gestures to help them settle. With this superpower comes a vulnerability to the trauma-experiences of others. As I have said above, this is particularly important for therapists who listen to many trauma stories. One therapist wrote:

I had just started working as a community health counsellor when a young man attended wanting help with his responses to a recent car accident. The accident had occurred just over a week ago. I asked him to outline what had happened. I realised afterwards that he plunged straight into a flashback, an intense recollection of the event. Although he drew a small diagram to show me where the car had been on the road, he was actively

> *re-experiencing the event. It happened so quickly and I was so new to the work that I didn't know what I was seeing or I would have helped him ground back into the moment in the session where he was safe. Instead, for five minutes, he described the accident in detail. No one was injured, but it was an almost catastrophic near-miss. In the moment of re-telling, he was terrified. As he spoke, I had an experience I haven't had since. Seeing and hearing him, I began to feel warmth in my body and face as though I had just had the sort of massive adrenalin rush you would experience in an accident. Like my client, I found myself sweating. After the session I found myself trembling and exhausted, like I had been hit by a truck, in this case literally and metaphorically. For a moment, on getting into my car at the end of the day, I experienced a wave of those feelings again. After that moment, the physical sensations left. The crucial point here is that I had not had the traumatic experience myself and had none of the visual memories, but close proximity to someone re-experiencing acute terror was in some way contagious for some elements of the experience.*

As the story above illustrates, vicarious trauma affects individual therapists. It can also affect organisations that work with trauma. The effects are often subtle and unacknowledged but nonetheless problematic. Another therapist wrote:

> *At one point I worked for a government organisation caring for people with intellectual disabilities. Our team of psychologists provided assessments of intellectual functioning that people needed to be able to access services. Part of the diagnosis of intellectual disability is that cognitive and behavioural deficits have been present since the early developmental period. It was a routine part of our work to draw out from individuals and families their stories of in-utero difficulties, birth injuries including those related to lack of oxygen, diagnoses, disabilities and illnesses present at birth or immediately afterwards, and the early signs of autism and other delays. This work had a significant effect on the mostly young women in our team. When we were contemplating having a family, pregnant, approaching*

> *delivery or raising young children, we had elevated anxiety about the possibility of something going wrong. Although the instances of such peri-natal difficulties are statistically low, our work made these risks particularly salient to us and produced an increased sense of our vulnerability to this sort of harm, a harm that in our world, at least, was over represented and vividly present to us.*

Vicarious trauma operates in many and varied ways in organisations. One of these is around the management of risk. Organisations that work with people—and especially vulnerable people—tend to receive much appropriate scrutiny. This is expressed across the organisation though such practices as the screening of staff, the provision of induction information, the shape of policies and day-to-day practices, and opportunities for feedback from clients and families. Risk is policed, as it were, from the top down. Government ministers, wanting very much to avoid crises on their watch, and the possibility of humiliating media coverage and demotion, inevitably convey down the line a degree of risk aversion and anxiety. Risk is discussed regularly at all levels of the organisation, often along with stories of failures and sanctions. At the level of the individual worker, tasks are monitored through supervision and also through casenotes.

Now obviously this sort of accountability is absolutely necessary. The challenge for organisations, leaders, and individuals, is how to hold the anxiety associated with risk in a way that is healthy and does not add to the anxiety within the organisational culture or to the anxiety of the practitioners actually working with clients. Done badly, everyone is stressed—often very well-meaning but stressed. Senior managers do not effectively contain the anxiety of the manager above them, and instead convey it further down the organisational ladder. Almost everyone, then, feels some sense of not being trusted, or some fear of reprimand or of losing their job, as a consequence of failures in this area. Done well, organisations are alert to this possibility, ensure very good processes, and encourage a strong culture of working within the processes. Risk management becomes a shared focus for the whole organisation, that is talked about, and where participation and feedback are encouraged. There is a culture of responsibility and trust, where managers are resourced to handle anxiety, and all front-line staff have independent clinical supervision. There is an organisation-wide culture that celebrates achievement and hard work and that recognises staff wellbeing as a priority and resource. At a surface level, organisations that are handling risk poorly or well may look quite similar. On the ground though, their emotional tones are very different.

As you will have noted from the stories above, vicarious trauma has a significant impact on the wellbeing of therapists. While such impacts could happen to any of us, there are some therapists who are at increased risk. There are factors that make it more likely that an individual who experiences a trauma will develop PTSD. These include pre-existing mental health conditions, exposure to prior traumatic experiences, and previous PTSD, and also experiencing traumas where other people are involved. These risk factors are obviously relevant for therapists, and it is likely they apply, as well, to the risk of vicarious trauma.

In addition, your own trauma history and any recent traumas you have experienced will be relevant in multiple ways to how you handle and respond to the trauma stories of clients. Almost inevitably, client stories that remind you of your own stories or their emotional content will affect you emotionally, and the trauma coping styles you have learnt will affect how you communicate with clients and respond to their specific trauma coping styles.

As well, the amount of exposure you have to trauma and the trauma stories of others is likely to affect your risk of vicarious trauma. Both these factors—your own history and the amount of trauma work you do—are particular areas of vulnerability for a subset of therapists. There is a dynamic that happens where people who have grown up with parents who were experiencing mental health issues or in neighbourhoods and communities where trauma was present, are drawn to helping professions. There are many strengths to this, including motivation and energy, but it also means that many caring professionals already have exposure to trauma before they commence this sort of work. As noted in 'Chapter 2: Know Yourself and Your History,' some therapists unconsciously choose work involving trauma as a form of trauma re-enactment, or as an opportunity for 'trauma mastery'. In addition to the other risks of such patterns, they are unwittingly increasing their already elevated trauma exposure, and thereby increasing their chances of both vicarious trauma and PTSD.

Suggestions

As always, bring trauma work to clinical supervision.

Be alert to both any vulnerability in your personal or work history, and the immediate impact of trauma content, so that you can continue your work with clients effectively but also debrief and apply self-care after sessions.

If you are not already familiar with *psychological first aid*, look up what this involves. It will be helpful for you and your clients.

If you have a trauma history yourself and haven't already done so, consider the Suggestions in Chapter 2.

Like other helping and medical professionals, therapists are often reluctant to seek out help for themselves. If you suspect you might be experiencing vicarious trauma, or that your work might be triggering past trauma or PTSD, please reach out for professional mental health support yourself.

Judith Herman writes with deep experience of the impact of trauma on the therapeutic relationship and on the therapist. Her take-home message is that therapists should only do this work with a support network around them. If this area is new to you, or one where you feel you need extra knowledge, I recommend chapter 7 of her *Trauma and Recovery: The aftermath of violence—From domestic abuse to political terror* (1992). If you are interested in how to look after yourself as you work with people experiencing trauma, and how to recognise and own the impact of your own trauma history on your choice to work in this field, I recommend *Trauma Stewardship: An everyday guide to caring for self while caring for others* (2009), by Laura Van Dernoot-Lipsky. Finally, in her book, *Help for the Helper: Preventing compassion fatigue and vicarious trauma in an ever-changing world* (2023), Babette Rothschild provides detailed practical steps for avoiding compassion fatigue and vicarious trauma. I recommend this most recent edition.

Workplace Tips

Organisations have an important role in both limiting the risk of vicarious trauma and helping workers who are affected by it. If an organisation acknowledges the risk to its staff, it will be more likely to provide regular and supportive supervision, to foster strong peer support, to provide regular trauma training, and to help staff to negotiate a balance in their work load so that they are not always working with traumatic content and have a measure of diversity in their caseload. Such organisations will also be more likely to acknowledge and validate a worker's experience of vicarious trauma when this occurs and to offer support services and adjustments to help with recovery.

Moral injury

The term Moral Injury was originally used to describe a type of enduring hurt that may occur to someone following a high-pressure, high-stakes, and potentially life-threatening situation where they have either acted in a way that violates their most deeply-held values or witnessed such acts and felt complicit. It was coined to describe the experience of people in military service who had killed or observed this happening, or heard repeated accounts of this happening, including in situations that might have involved harm to women and children, and where it was difficult to distinguish civilians or where protecting civilians was against orders. Common responses included guilt, shame, embarrassment, anger, contempt, disgust, and disillusionment with and disconnection from a sense of humanity.

Initially, the aim of the label Moral Injury seems to have been to normalise or de-pathologise the responses of individuals and to convey that moral anguish is a normal response to abnormal situations. Based on the description above, many of these military personnel had also been exposed to circumstances that would put them at risk of PTSD. Given the high prevalence of PTSD among service personnel, it is tempting to say that PTSD too is a normal response to abnormal circumstances, or at very least, a common response. There are benefits though to the label Moral Injury. It may help explain the responses of people who do not otherwise meet criteria for PTSD, and it serves to highlight a particular type of struggle experienced by people with PTSD.

Apparently one of the hopes of the original proponents of the term was to highlight and explore treatments for issues like shame and guilt that were not well addressed by other approaches to PTSD. Now, at one level this is disappointing, as trauma-focussed CBT for PTSD, Exposure Therapy, and Cognitive Processing Therapy for PTSD may all involve extensive work on thinking patterns and associated emotions including guilt and shame. In addition, while it's true that much of this therapy work is focussed on victims, these therapies are also effective in work with people with PTSD who have perpetrated violence. It's possible, though, that potential clients in this second category avoid therapy, or withhold content about their own role, due to fear of social or legal repercussions, precisely when this is what is fuelling their symptoms. The term Moral Injury may provide a way of recognising and potentially addressing the harms that come to people who choose or feel compelled to act violently as part of their role and/or under circumstances of extreme threat.

Another aspect of the term that I appreciate is the way it highlights the potential origins of this injury, in deeply-held values. I wonder if the reason that some people receiving therapy for PTSD— even the therapies above—have not found them helpful for guilt and shame, is that the related thought patterns may be easily evaluated and dismissed by secular therapists, when their less-secular clients may need to have these issues, often grounded in religious, spiritual, and moral beliefs, taken seriously.

This insight into and reminder of the role of deeply-held values in trauma and recovery has relevance for how we think of the impact of trauma on our clients. It can be helpful to think of a continuum, with moral injury at the far end of a continuum of moral and ethical harms, moral distress, moral frustration and moral challenge. Some of the most debilitating cases of PTSD I have seen have been in civilian clients— usually women—who were previously in violent relationships where there was much emotional coercion beside. In that context of coercion, though not necessarily under the threat of immediate harm or injury, they were induced by their partners to engage in sexual behaviours they themselves regarded as shameful and humiliating. They are usually extremely reluctant to reveal this part of their story, fearing even more judgement, alongside their own self-recriminations. As a result, this material and the thoughts they have about themselves often go unchallenged and without healing. I suspect that these cases bear some relationship to the idea of moral injury, more broadly defined.

There may also be some element of vicarious moral injury present for therapists sitting with clients whose experience of use-and-abuse has left them negative about life and society in general. I have encountered families that have experienced several generations of child sexual abuse, undisclosed, largely unacknowledged or denied, and without serious consequences for perpetrators. Often even the adult victims are somewhat hopeless about their ability to make a difference or to keep the next generation safe. It is as though their moral set point for hopefulness has been damaged. In the face of the injury that has happened to their clients' moral ground and capacity for hope, the therapist needs to be resilient in their own personal counter-narrative or they may be at risk of hopelessness themselves.

The terms Moral Distress and Moral Injury have been applied to groups beyond miliary service personnel, including health care workers and emergency responders, such as firefighters and police. In these circumstances, the distress is understood to arise in situations of ethical conflict, where the right course of action is clear but is made nearly impossible due to organisational processes and limitations. Specifically, it is suggested that the experience of being unable to provide sufficient care in life-threatening circumstances may result in Moral Injury. This was a situation faced by many front-line health care workers in the worst moments of the COVID-19 pandemic.

Defined in this way, as a distress arising in the gaps between what seems right and what is possible, where the circumstances are life-threatening, it seems likely that if not Moral Injury as this term was originally intended, then that at very least a form of moral stress may be relevant to the experience of some therapists. Even when governments provide funding to support therapy, there are often lengthy waiting lists, and many clients who cannot afford gap fees or for whom funded sessions are grossly inadequate. These are often the clients with histories of chronic and complex trauma, starting from childhood, and as we noted earlier, for many of these clients their mental health conditions result in life-threatening behaviours.

In addition to this lack of available sessions, which can at least be partially attributed to government and client decisions, or organisational policy, there is the challenge to therapists presented by our therapies themselves and the limits to which they are effective. We can see that our therapies could be effective, but in practice there are barriers and limits, including in how we deliver the therapies. In this context, perhaps therapists with high standards and self-sacrificing self-concepts have an increased vulnerability to moral harm, or something like it.

As well, there may be a risk for therapists of moral harm in repeatedly hearing stories—from abusers and the abused—about adults behaving badly to children or other adults in ways that violate the therapist's most deeply held values. I am thinking of the many stories therapists hear both of physical and sexual abuse from carers to children, and also of emotional abuse, such as continual indifference, denigration or hostility. When listening to some of the more extreme stories, it is possible to tell ourselves that the child protection system is continually improving and that such cases would now be prevented. We know, however, that so many cases are never reported and that many others, particularly of emotional abuse, happen in what families takes to be the normal course of life and rarely attract the attention of someone who might protest and act to protect the child. In addition, our government child protection systems are so busy that only the most severe cases receive attention and the interactions of families with the child protection services often make very little positive difference. The psychological and social challenges families face are often very complicated and are so often further compounded by social and economic disadvantage. Although there may be some government money available for early intervention, it is hardly enough. While often labelled a priority by governments at election times, families are largely left to their own devices.

And then there are the deep limitations of many 'out of home' care situations for children. While there is the temptation to think that if a given client had been taken out of their emotionally abusive context they would have been spared further harm, the now generations of people who have been in out of home residential care, attest the risks involved and the negative effects on attachment.

Questions that arise for therapists may include why our societies, and the governments they elect, condone these situations or are unwilling or unable to offer different policies or procedures. In these circumstances, a therapist may come to lose hope in their society's ability to raise children well enough and safely. Rather than an acute disillusionment with and disconnection from a sense of shared humanity, this may be more gradual and subtle. I suspect that advocates for asylum-seekers locked up indefinitely and therapists and community support-staff working with groups experiencing intergenerational trauma struggle similarly.

Suggestions

The moral challenges of therapy work, while rarely discussed, are numerous and can be debilitating. If this is an unfamiliar topic for you, consider reading a little more on the topic. Therapists who are affected in these ways need to draw on all that they know about self-care. In addition, this is one of several areas where self-care will ideally draw on a therapist's own deep values and resources, including the values that have previously motivated their work. If this mention of deep values and resources interests you, keep reading. Giving and receiving support among colleagues can be helpful. Using your best judgement, consider spending time with people who share your deeply-held values. One challenge here can be that non-therapist supporters are generally not familiar with the many barriers to good care that exist in the day-to-day lives of clients. For that reason, it can be particularly helpful to meet with other therapists who share your interests or concerns and who are seeking to advocate. Many larger professional bodies have interest groups of this kind. If there isn't one in existence, and you cannot find like-minded and engaged therapists online through more informal social media networks, consider starting a network of your own.

Finally, if you find moral distress continuing or you have reason to think you are also experiencing post-trauma symptoms or even PTSD, please reach out for professional support.

Workplace Tips

Many of the strategies that are helpful in reducing the risk of vicarious trauma and supporting staff who are affected, are relevant for Moral Injury and related harms. The document, *Moral Stress Amongst Healthcare Workers During COVID-19: A Guide to Moral Injury*, developed by Phoenix Australia – Centre for Posttraumatic Mental Health and the Canadian Centre of Excellence – PTSD, contains specific recommendations for individuals, organisations, and team leaders. While the context for the document was the COVID-19 pandemic, the information about moral injury and related harms and the suggestions it offers are relevant more broadly.

Take-home message:

Transference and countertransference, vicarious trauma, and moral injury have significant deleterious effects on the work of many therapists. To reduce your risk of therapist disenchantment and to support yourself when you have been negatively affected, do what you can to inform yourself about how they operate, to develop practices for noticing and reflection, and to get extra support in the form of both an ongoing network and, when needed, specific mental health treatment.

Where to next?

We move now to the penultimate section of the book, looking at the range of professional and organisational challenges that therapists encounter. The next chapter looks in detail at the demands of our organisational settings and professional contexts.

CHAPTER 5

Context is Everything

In Australia, the national government currently provides funding for psychology sessions directly to appropriately registered individual practitioners. That funding is available under government legislation and with many limits and expectations, not all of which are easily available for reference. The legislation and the policies by which the legislation is applied are also frequently updated. This type of funding arrangement can readily produce confusion and anxiety, particularly in already overworked, time-poor therapists. I recall that when I first started working as a consultant under these arrangements, one colleague talked in nightmare-inducing terms about how, if we were audited by our funding body, incorrect wording on a client referral from a general family medical practitioner could result in the funding body demanding money back. She said this had happened to a colleague of hers and that it had ruined her business and life. As you can imagine, this increased my already elevated new-practitioner-stress.

This is, of course, a very specific example of one of the many and varied ways that our organisational settings and professional context can affect us as therapists. In this chapter, we will take a brief tour of some of the layers of context in which we work, and the challenges and opportunities they offer. I invite you to reflect on your own layers of context and to consider which elements might be contributing to your stress, distress or disenchantment. The final section then includes some practical suggestions for navigating these contexts and some ideas for how to make the most of the resources you have available.

Layers of context

I invite you to imagine your layers of professional context as a series of concentric circles. Even as I describe them, perhaps you might draw something similar, in whatever form would work for you. Although aspects of our professional context, like governmental and legislative influence, work across circles, this model of concentric circles has the immediate virtue of helping us to hold in mind many aspects of context at the same time.

The inner circle represents you and your immediate family, and your need for income to resource the things that matter to you. This circle includes your guiding needs, hopes, values, and goals in relation to work.

One layer out is your immediate work context, team, unit or program. As therapists we work in private practices of many varieties, religious congregations, publicly-funded hospitals and services, privately-funded organisations, and community-funded services, and this list will inevitably miss other contexts. Perhaps you work in a private practice for others as a contractor, or for yourself, or in a partnership, or where you employ or contract others to work for you? Or perhaps you work in an organisation where you draw a salary. In that immediate workplace context, wherever it is, consider all the people to whom you answer. It could be simply your clients. You may have employees. You may have managers above you and people who report to you or who you manage or supervise. In addition to your roles, you may note here the many and varied relationships you have with colleagues and peers and the expectations that come with those interpersonal relationships.

Beyond your immediate work context, there are other layers of context. If you are in a private practice, these might be third-party funding providers or community groups to whom you advertise, or who have an interest in your work, or service providers who clean your offices, or from whom you hire your premises. If you work in a unit within a larger organisation, there may be other levels of context still, including expectations, named and unnamed, from more senior levels of the organisation. The larger organisation will also exist within a network of stakeholders, funding providers, and community interests.

Beyond these layers you might belong to voluntary professional bodies or associations. In addition, you may be formally registered with one or more professional bodies, which are part of the broader health regulatory environment.

The different levels of government influence within which you work are also important context, starting from your local council, and including any regional or state governments, and your national government.

For completeness, it is worth adding to these layers one for your national context and another for your international or global context.

Challenges and opportunities

While some of the layers I mentioned above may usually be some distance from your thinking, I suspect that some immediately stood out as current sources of stress or concern for you. If you can, take a moment to note those areas and concerns. We will return to them.

Without presenting a comprehensive summary, this section highlights some of the challenges and opportunities that arise for therapists at these various layers. I have two aims here. The first is to help you identify other less immediate pressures and concerns that are affecting your work and that you might want to address. The second is to stimulate your thinking about the balance between demands and resources in these areas and whether there are resources present that might be worth considering.

Let's start with work in private practice. There are tremendous appeals to working for yourself, in setting the tone and creating procedures for yourself. There are also huge challenges to working for yourself, where everything rests on you, including the income you generate. You are the person who must navigate fee payment with clients and obligations with third party funders. While some therapists worked from home long before our experience of a global pandemic, as this became an almost universal experience for office workers for several years, most of us now understand in a much more personal way the challenges and vulnerabilities that can come with physical and professional isolation. Some of the many that come to mind include the temptation to overwork, the difficulties of separating work from the rest of life, and the reduced opportunities to debrief and access alternate perspectives.

As a small business owner with contracted therapists and one or more paid staff, you have much greater autonomy than someone working in a large organisation, but everything also rests on you, including finding the information you need, generating enough income, or being sufficiently organised to arrange for contractors or employees to bring in the income. Writing about their experience, one therapist told me:

A small business where I was a contracting private psychologist attempted an experiment. They had had difficulty recruiting contracting psychologists. They offered several salaried positions based on seeing 25 clients a week. On the surface this was reasonable. After all, some of the more unscrupulous centres insist that contractors see seven to eight clients or more a day. As well, the proposed income for general psychologists was about what they would have earnt if they had been doing those hours as a private practitioner, but it came with the assurance of a wage and basic benefits. The owner was seeking a reliable workforce, at minimal cost. Contractors are all very well, but they pick and choose their own days and hours, and over time she had come to think of them as an unreliable source of labour. Unfortunately, the plan was shaky from the start. Clients often didn't turn up, so through no fault of their own the new staff couldn't meet their targets. They overbooked and became exhausted. With that volume of client work, they needed a lot of clinical supervision, which wasn't always available. They quickly discovered that it takes many hours to administer client hours, what with preparation, creating resources, follow-up, and report-writing. To administer five days of clients, or 25 clients, probably takes two further days. So, it turned out that a modestly paid job was requiring 50 plus hours to complete, not factoring in the significant emotional impact of seeing that number of clients a week. Most experienced practitioners in private practice find it hard to sustain a full client load for four days a week, in any ongoing way. None of the new staff lasted two years and the majority left with a degree of discontent toward the owner. Their discontent was only matched by that of the business practitioner-owner, frustrated that one more attempt to do something about her extremely slim business margins had failed.

As a contractor or an employee in a company, especially a smaller company, you will certainly have a considerable degree of autonomy, but with that is often a degree of professional isolation, as you and your fellow contractors pass each other briefly in the hallway, but rarely have time and space to build community. If you are very fortunate, there may be peer supervision available in your organisation. In this context, you are to some extent vulnerable to the company's decisions about whether to comply with professional ethical standards and external reporting requirements. Particularly as a contractor, you will be individually responsible for developing many of your own processes, providing care to clients, and answering if something goes wrong, but it can be difficult from that position to know whether your organisation has good practices, or to believe you can influence those decisions. Often, as well, contractor therapists find there is limited variety in their work, and almost no scope to change roles within their organisations. The only paths to greater variety may be to re-train at their own expense or to take the leap to another type of workplace.

On the other hand, perhaps you work as a therapist within a section of a much larger organisation. As you might expect, there are pluses and minuses to this situation. There may be myriad expectations, processes, and procedures surrounding how your work is completed, and these may change on a regular basis, and have significant implications for how you do your work. You may have limited influence on those processes and how they are developed or implemented. Common challenges for counsellors and therapists in this setting are the number of clients they are expected to see each day and the number of sessions they are allowed to have with individual clients. On the other side of the ledger, with some form of human resources and payroll structure in place, there is an increased chance that you will have paid clinical supervision, a predictable income, and additional legislated benefits including employer contributions to your pension, superannuation or social security, holiday pay, sick pay and so on.

Perhaps you are in a senior therapist role that involves providing therapy, supervision, and management. This comes with the benefits of variety and income, and the privilege and power to shape a future generation of therapists. The challenges of such positions, however, are in the volume of work, the increasing difficulty you may have in locating a trusted clinical supervisor or peer mentor for your own work, and in the tensions that may arise due to role conflicts and boundary issues where your workplace asks you to provide both clinical and management supervision to staff.

Whatever your workplace setting or level of seniority as a therapist, you will also be negotiating the essentials of most workplaces: Who are my clients? How do I care for my clients in this context? Beyond my clients, to whom do I report or have obligations? How do I meet the stated and unstated expectations of my work context? How do I communicate, negotiate, and establish relationships with my superiors and my juniors? How do I want to contribute to the culture and tone of this workplace? How do I manage my frustrations and disappointments when things don't go smoothly in these areas or colleagues behave badly? And, how will I respond to the frustrations and disappointments of those around me?

In-between your immediate workplace and any government context, there may well be other stakeholders you need to consider. Perhaps your primary funding comes through health insurers regulated by government but acting also in the profit-interests of their companies. Or perhaps you are registered with a number of different agencies that send clients to therapy. In Australia, as example, there are pools for funding available through Workcover, the Traffic Accident Commission, the National Disability Insurance Scheme, and various state-based victims of crime support programs. This doesn't include the various Employee Assistance Programs, large and small.

While such arrangements bring with them extra income streams, the costs may include the time and money needed to register and then comply with reporting and billing requirements. Even though there is funding available, its availability also highlights the rules around its provision. Certain services can be provided to certain people and not to others. Sometimes this is frustrating and sometimes it seems ridiculous or even unjust. Sometimes the ways funding is provided also cause divisions between colleagues, as some receive more than others. Being dependent on funding also brings with it, at times, a level of powerlessness. If the government or funding body does not want to review funding arrangements, or make increases in line with the Consumer Price Index, a therapist or organisation may have little recourse except to tighten their belts or find other sources of funding.

Voluntary professional bodies come with other sets of related but distinct benefits and demands. There are fees, expectations about professional behaviour, and possible snobberies about who is in and who is out. There are the benefits, including digested information about changes to the work context—the legislative and regulatory contexts already mentioned—opportunities to network, and access to professional development resources.

While these organisations provide information, they also represent vested interests that determine what is filtered through to members. This can feel frustrating. In these days of social media, there are many additional and sometimes even alternative sources of information and support. They, of course, have their own vested interests, and are more or less well funded and credible.

There are definite benefits that come from some sort of registration, including the ability to claim particular sorts of funding, and the knowledge that your professional group is generally well-regarded by the community. There are, on the other hand, the financial costs of registration, and the expectations about what is required to obtain and maintain registration, and what it means to comply with professional standards of behaviour.

An associated challenge for therapists is the sheer volume of information that exists in legislation and regulation, or that comes in emails and journals from registration and professional bodies. Those expectations also come with demands on my time to record things and complete paperwork. In the gap between the volume of that information and my capacity to read and absorb it, I have frequently experienced anxiety about whether I am complying and whether there will be negative consequences when I fail to do so.

As a counter-balance, I've come to understand that many—although not all—expectations by our professional bodies, actually represent attempts to codify important elements of standard professional care. Professional expectations are generally very helpful pointers and guides. Codes of ethics and guidelines for professional conduct, while coming with expectations, also represent a great deal of accumulated experience about how to navigate the sometimes-rocky shoals of human interaction. Professional emails and journals often locate and synthesise huge volumes of information that individual practitioners would find it hard or even impossible to locate and digest. They provide information about professional development and networking opportunities that are important in the often very isolated world of therapists. However unwieldy and opaque professional bodies can appear at times, they often also provide a larger and more resourced base from which to advocate for change than that of an individual practitioner, workplace, or online interest group.

Moving on, you might consider what if any challenges and benefits come to you as a therapist through the various levels of government: local, regional, state and national. Known and unknown, you will have responsibilities outlined in legislation, statutes, and bylaws. At a very practical level, if you are a small business owner, your local council's decisions will inevitably affect you, whether they are about fees for rubbish removal, or what types of business can occur in particular areas. Of more pressing concern perhaps, in many countries one or more levels of government determine which therapists can be employed or funded and to what extent. These decisions are made with varying degrees of consultation with clients, communities, mental health researchers, service providers, and their professional associations. There will be benefits, of course, to operating within all these layers of government, including a more or less predictable business environment, possible sources of funding, and a structure in which to seek justice, if something isn't working and can't be resolved. Of course, depending on where in the world you are reading this, the benefits provided by government to your work as a therapist may be less obvious and their expectations and decisions seemingly more capricious.

For a moment, consider the impact of your nation's situation within a community of nations on your therapy practice. Is your country currently experiencing internal or external peace or conflict? How is it viewed internationally? Due to war, or economic hardship, or internal conflict, has your country become a departure point for migrants and refugees or, instead, is it seen as an attractive destination?

Finally, and for completeness, consider the impact of international and global trends and issues on your own life, the lives of your clients, and on your work together. Examples might include the proliferation of personal digital devices and the ubiquity of social media platforms, the consequences of widespread diseases or events impacting global finances, and the outcomes of climate change.

There are at least three levels at which this context affects us. It intersects with those personal patterns and ways of being in the world we have acknowledged, including our histories and health. In addition, there are the practical constraints and demands of the work. As well, there are the ways these emotional, cognitive, and practical demands balance with the resources we have available. This balance of demands and resources is very important. Where the demands are too great for the resources available, we may begin to experience strain and even discontentment. I suspect that most of us are not surprised that it is the pressures of this broader context that often prompt therapists to leave their work. If you want to continue your work as a therapist, you will need to find a path where the balance of demands to resources is lifegiving for you.

Suggestions

If you haven't already done so, create some way of representing these layers of context for your work. Note down the good things about different aspects of your work context. This is important, because these benefits can be valuable resources. Note down also the areas where you are aware of stresses or concerns.

I recommend a structured problem-solving approach. List the key areas from this review that represent a problem and then pick the most pressing area for attention. In the space of an A4 page, in three columns, allow yourself to brainstorm options and solutions and then to acknowledge the pluses and minuses of each option. Do not limit yourself to tried and true options and solutions, but allow for as many others as you can, including more fanciful ones, like your equivalent of my own, 'move to Barbados'. Consider also ways you might use the good things about your work context to address these problems. There is power in taking the time to write these options down and to acknowledge the pluses and minuses. We often do this process by mental short-hand, without acknowledging the actual constraints upon us, the reasons we have been doing things the way we have to this point, and the potential areas of choice open to us. Get it all out on paper or on your screen. Then choose the best option or two and implement them. Make sure though that you then review whether and how this worked for you. Perhaps your plan needs a minor modification or perhaps it needs to be thrown out completely and replaced by one of the other options on the list. See how this works for your most pressing item and then, if needed, move on to the second most pressing item. Our workplace issues are often complicated and multifaceted. That said, though, our basic therapy tools often work just as well for us as they do for our clients.

In addition, and as you would expect by now, I encourage you to have some regular way of reflecting on your work, rather than finding yourself routinely reacting. If your workplace clinical supervision is sufficiently independent to allow space to discuss these questions, take full advantage of it. If you need more clinical supervision or a supervisor with greater independence from the workplace, or even a therapist, do what you can to arrange that, even if only for a few sessions, as the need arises. In some countries you may be able to claim supervision as a tax deduction as a cost incurred in the process of earning income.

If you are an early-career therapist or quite new in your workplace, and experiencing anxiety about all you do not know, remind yourself that you generally don't need to know everything all at once. In a new work context, it helps tremendously to have a competent management supervisor, regular clinical supervision, and also reliable and experienced colleagues who can distil information to you and pass on their knowledge of responsible and professional processes. If you don't know such people, do what you can to locate them and to find reliable people who can guide you.

As you can, develop routines for reading workplace and professional emails and journals, and ways to gather and save therapy resources and professional information so that you can find them again when needed.

If you are developing a private practice, consider creating therapy resources of your own, rather than relying on others to provide resources. For example, professional bodies often provide templates for consent procedures and, if you need them, these can be modified to suit your context. The cost in the time it takes you to locate the templates and then to modify them will be repaid many times over in the confidence you have that you are operating within a sound client consent structure. Similarly, over time, learn how to record your business finances, and how to introduce clients to the therapy process. Find ways of recording what you communicate to clients, what sessions you have, and what correspondence you have sent and for what reasons. Locate assessment frameworks and modify them. Gather, create, and modify resources for clients, including emergency and 24-hour support numbers, short-term and first aid emotional support resources, and medium-to-long-term therapy resources. You will notice that many of these resources, while on the one hand meeting various professional expectations about consent, confidentiality, and record-keeping, are also resources for the therapeutic relationship itself and for the client. It takes time to build up such resources, though, and you will need to practice a degree of patience with yourself about the gaps between what you know and do in these areas and what you *might* know and do. Over time, if you continue your journey as a therapist, you will acquire knowledge, experience, and wisdom about what most needs attention and what can wait.

Finally, use your therapy knowledge to manage your own responses, and if you need extra skills in this area, you can be confident that any time you invest in personal development will strengthen your work as a therapist. As specific examples, anything you learn about management and organisational skills, higher-level communication and assertiveness skills, about working fruitfully with others, and about your own values and motivations, will improve your experience of work, now and in the future.

Workplace Tip

If you are in a position to influence decision-making in your workplace, consider surveying staff about workplace successes and pressures, and inviting problem-solving suggestions from across all levels of the organisation.

Take-home message:

Pressures from our workplace context regularly contribute to therapist disenchantment and often prompt therapists to move jobs or leave their work. If you want to continue your work as a therapist, you will need to find ways to navigate these pressures. As a starting point, review your current circumstances and consider who might be available to support you.

Where to next?

Two chapters follow on professional crises and how to handle them.

CHAPTER 6

When Things Go to Hell in a Handbasket, or How to Handle Professional Crises

Professional crises

At some couple counselling training I attended we were told that most couples who stay in their relationship will have about five crises. Whether you wanted them or not, the crises were coming. In order to stay together, couples had to find a way of negotiating crises. I believe similar things are true about our relationship to our work as therapists if we are to continue lifegiving and fruitful work with clients. We should expect and prepare for crises in our relationship to our work, be these related to the stage of our lives and careers, or to the unexpected. This chapter introduces some of the most common professional crises, and discusses two specifically: taking on too much client work too soon, whether as a young or beginning therapist or when starting a new job, and burnout.

There is no clear line between professional and personal crises, of course, and some crises fit into both categories. Businesses burn down or are flooded. Companies that employ therapists unexpectedly go out of business. Sometimes the community in which a therapist is living is affected by disease, natural disaster, or civil, military or political unrest. In these circumstances, therapists find themselves having to survive and adjust personally and professionally, while supporting others going through similar things. Our global experience of the COVID-19 pandemic has been such an experience, and one where, in addition to personal and professional adjustments, the number of people seeking mental health support has increased substantially, adding further pressures to an already difficult situation. In this respect, the experience of therapists shares something with that of front-line healthcare workers, teachers, and other essential workers during this global emergency. Many in these groups have been pained by the gaps between the care they would like to provide to others and what seems possible in their settings. Many have wondered at times, 'Who cares for the carer?' We have seen, in the large number of resignations from these roles in recent times, an answer to this question. In situations where the demands on individuals continue to outstrip their capacity and the available resources, they may choose to leave roles that were hard-won and previously meaningful.

One of the most stressful events a therapist can experience is the death by suicide of a current client. That is probably followed closely by the death by suicide of a client you have seen in the previous year. Both may well mean that you need to prepare a report for the coroner about your work with the deceased client. At about the same level of stress would be learning that your files or accounts are to be audited, or that a complaint has been made about your work to your professional registration body, or that you are being subpoenaed to appear in court to give evidence or speak in regard to a report you have written. These situations tend to be more stressful still when you have some cause to think your behaviour was not all you wish it had been. We make mistakes, of course, and it doesn't usually result in professional suspension or deregistration. It may involve a public or private reprimand though, and as adults, this is territory most of us very much want to avoid. Such complaints, and any reprimand or sanction, are likely to trigger our existing schemas, be they high standards, defectiveness, mistrust, or negativity and pessimism, and none of us want to experience professional humiliation, loss of income, loss of a job, or reduced chances of employment in the future.

One of the risks for therapists in facing such challenges is that we often work alone. Therapists who work from home rather than in clinics, and pastoral workers who are in small communities with no other pastors nearby, are similarly at risk due to isolation. This makes us vulnerable to all those unhelpful thinking patterns we encountered in Chapter One. In addition, therapists themselves are not always kind to other therapists. Our high standards, or our desire to avoid our own feelings of vulnerability, can often result in critical, dismissive, and even contemptuous behaviour toward other therapists. Perhaps you recognise yourself in this description. If you have been a therapist for any length of time, you will have encountered such behaviour in colleagues. Such experiences do not encourage transparent and healthy workplaces or practices. Neither do they encourage supportive collegial relationships. Most of us have learnt that if a peer can be destructively critical of someone else, they can be similarly critical of us.

Suggestions

At all times, make sure you are appropriately registered and insured.

In advance of any professional crises, know your code of ethics and the relevant legislation around your work. If you are not familiar with how to respond to subpoenas or the implications for privacy and confidentiality, check the website for your professional body or speak to an experienced colleague. Try to keep this area on your list of potential professional development activities, even if only in the form of some occasional reading.

Talk about issues of ethical practice regularly with your clinical supervisor and make a note in your supervision records of any specific client issues you discussed and any outcomes or recommendations.

Always work within the limits of your competence and with an eye to recency of practice—that is, keeping in mind how recently you have refreshed your knowledge about a topic and worked with clients with the same problem or something very similar. This is as important in the later part of your career as it is in the early part.

Over time, build up an understanding about good and safe practice. Learn from the experience of colleagues and from your own experience.

If you possibly can, work on your professional networks across your career. Do what you can to build up long-term and trusted connections. Make such connections your priority. Such networks are one of many resources that can keep you at work as a therapist and they are meaningful ways that you can also be a support to colleagues.

Many professional bodies have an advice line for members facing ethical and legal challenges, and some forms of professional indemnity insurance come with free hours of legal advice. If you can, before any such crises emerge, know how to access these resources.

If all else fails, though, and your client dies, or one of these other crises emerges, find a colleague you respect. If the first one doesn't meet you where you are, find a second one. Get support. Locate one or more experienced colleagues who can journey with you, be this your clinical supervisor or someone else. If you are being supervised specifically for registration or a specialised qualification, then your clinical supervisor will need to know. If they can't help you with a particular crisis, they should be able to refer to you a colleague for some additional support.

If you know you sometimes fall into the trap of criticising colleagues, think about the sort of response and care you would want to receive in such a crisis.

Too much too soon, or 'Perhaps I'm not cut out for this work'

You may either have been this therapist or can immediately think of a colleague in this situation: On the strength of completing his qualification and professional registration, he has decided to hang up his own shingle and establish a full-time private practice. In Australia, appropriately trained psychologists in private practice are funded by the government and the demand for psychological care almost always outstrips supply. Or, perhaps this young therapist has been fortunate enough to secure full-time clinical work in the community or in government. Whatever the context, he suddenly finds himself with a full and varied caseload of clients. Not realising all the preparation and follow-up needed for each session, and the emotional and physical toll of the work, he has completely booked his days with clients.

Perhaps some of what he will later come to understand as *over*booking comes from a passion for helping, overconfidence, an attempt to prove his capacity or poorly considered financial commitments. Perhaps he is working for an organisation that routinely overloads new graduates for one reason or another. This is a common risk for young practitioners who first set up as contractors in the private sector, or employees of organisations that only receive fees when clients attend their clinics. Even caring practitioner-owners can lose sight of the impact on new staff of insisting that they see seven or more clients, day after day. Overload can also happen in community, education, and government roles where there is simply too much work for the staff available. In either case, though, if he is working for someone, it may be hard for this young or new practitioner to resist organisational pressures. If he is in private practice, it may be easier or harder for him to pull back hours himself, as that will depend on the factors that led him to set up private practice in the first place.

One of the things that young or new practitioners often miss is the amount of preparation and follow-up required for clients. In addition to the practical and administrative aspects of the work, including casenotes, early in your career or role, clients will present regularly with issues and diagnoses that are unfamiliar to you. This almost automatically causes a great deal of stress for beginning therapists who come to their roles with the desire to help and the expectation that they will be highly effective and know all the answers. An experienced lecturer of mine said that by the time you have been a therapist for five years, you have probably seen an example of most issues, but that it takes that long. He added, however, that it doesn't take that long to know how to run an effective first session. With very good training placements, or after a first year of full-time supervised practice, you may have that under your belt. For several years though, after that first session, you will often need to investigate what the research says about how to proceed and what resources that client might need. The same lecturer told us, 'You only need to be one session ahead of where you are with your client. In some situations, this will be unavoidable.' He helpfully described one situation when treating a client with an unfamiliar condition where he was in the session with the client, treatment manual on his knee.

The sort of time needed to prepare for sessions in this way doesn't include the time you need to debrief with a colleague, to make a follow-up call to a client's former therapist, or to call the emergency services to arrange a welfare check to the client over the weekend.

Neither does it include the physical and emotional impacts of the work. Sometimes young active therapists comment to me about all the sitting involved. It is certainly one of the hazards of the work. In addition, it is impossible for newly graduated practitioners to guess the emotional impact of the work. You cannot sit opposite clients most of the day, many of whom are experiencing intense emotional states, without it affecting you. It is enough for now to say that as a therapist you will need far more time for self-care than you first imagined.

Much of the burden of therapy arises from situations where clients are presenting with issues that are on the edge of—or beyond—both our professional skills and knowledge and our own journey's depth and scope. Most of the time, and especially for clients who haven't had much therapy, even a beginning therapist will have something to offer. Often though, as described above, a therapist may be only one session ahead. In early-to-mid-career, there is always a possibility that clients are wondering about or offering to open areas that the therapist is yet to work on for themselves. The therapist may either not acknowledge or hear them or actively avoid the material. More experienced therapists who recognise what is happening may be able to listen well enough to allow a client to go to places they themselves have not considered. This is one of many situations where therapists and clients may be genuinely co-explorers. For early career therapists, however, and especially where the mismatch between client needs and therapist capability is highest, there is a tremendous drain on therapist resources.

As a result of all these pressures, a fair proportion of young and new practitioners crash-and-burn in one form or another within a few months, and certainly within the first year. If they don't have wise counsel, or some option for flexibility in their work hours, they may find themselves very quickly headed toward burnout. Perhaps the most devastating outcome here is the impact on how young or new practitioners think about themselves and their suitability for the work. Those wounds can be hard to heal. If the picture I have painted sounds relevant to you, keep reading.

Suggestions

If you want to avoid this path altogether, or recognise the early signs of being on this journey, plan a break of at least a day but preferably a week. While on your break, if you don't already have one, develop your intentional self-care plan. Make sure the plan involves ways of being physically active around or outside work hours.

Book in more frequent sessions with your clinical supervisor. If you are a young or new therapist or new in your role, you probably need to see your clinical supervisor at least fortnightly. That bare minimum of clinical supervision once a month will not suffice. You will know you are having enough clinical supervision when your symptoms of stress reduce. Then you can gradually start to space out sessions again.

Be scrupulous about abiding by the ethical imperative to work within the limits of your competence. Find out which of your colleagues specialise in what areas, or how to find appropriately experienced colleagues in the local area, and refer your clients on as needed. This is not a failure on your part. Done well, it is the height of good practice.

Experiment with what the ideal number of client sessions is for you each day, given the number of days you are working. If you need to, and have the freedom to do so, experiment with what the ideal number of client days is for you across a week.

Become very good at your core work. Whatever your primary modality, whether you are a CBT-practitioner, Narrative or Solution-Focussed therapist, or something else, make it your first order of business to be skilled in that therapy. Eclectic practice may or may not come to you later. For now, though, become very good at using your primary therapy with a range of clients. Attend professional development training, watch quality and substantial online materials, and read the key texts by well-regarded practitioners and teachers of your therapy. Becoming skilled at your therapy is not just a matter of adding theoretical knowledge to what you learnt in your course. It involves learning in more detailed ways how to apply this theory to practice with individuals using individual treatment formulations. This is the heart of the art and science of therapy and can be a place of considerable satisfaction, as the work is created anew for each client.

As a stretch goal, get to know your ethical framework and the legislative and regulatory context in which you are paid. Difficulties in these areas often cause considerable anxiety for new therapists. The better you know the framework in which you work, the more secure you can be in your practice.

Finally, keep in mind that the 'too much, too soon' experience is not limited to young and new practitioners. It is a familiar experience for those of us who have started new roles, or who have changed roles within our field. Talking to a colleague about the idea for this book, she said, 'It happens so often. There was someone who worked here. She was very good with clients. You could see it from how they responded to her. Then she went for her clinical registration and was working all these hours and she just fell apart.' So, be alert for the signs of overload and kind to yourself if you notice them. One of the great benefits of experience is that you might be able to intervene earlier on your own behalf than you knew to do in the first years of your career.

Is this burnout?

My experience of the early stages of burnout happened when I worked in a high-volume customer service role, at the front desk of an office providing care to university students. The pace of the work was relentless, and particularly so at the beginning of semester. Arriving students, telephone calls, mail, and email, all needed to be answered as soon as possible. Often the front desk was several students deep and staffed only by one extra person. My immediate superior was friendly but did not seem to grasp the volume of the work. Like the rest of the office, she was under considerable pressure herself. The overall unit manager was a strong woman with a short-temper and a tendency to be punitive if disappointed. I had been punished for perceived failings and constantly felt like I was trying to prove myself. In this context, I gradually began to experience the stages of burnout, starting first with feeling very stressed and eventually moving to a persistent feeling of being overwhelmed, where I found it hard to concentrate. I began to have very negative thoughts about my workplace and my boss. On some occasions, I was so angry and tired that it was hard to be gracious to all the people turning up at the reception desk. As I was a junior staff member, and it was evident to me that I didn't have sufficient influence to change the work situation, I found another job. I was later told that when I left the workplace discovered they needed to employ several ongoing staff to cover the desk that had been staffed by me and some casually-employed students. For the first few days in my new role, I noticed the familiar dread and anxiety when I arrived. When this happened, I needed to remind myself that I was now in a different setting. Soon enough, as I experienced a normal workload and supportive and appreciative management, those symptoms of burnout settled.

This outcome points to one important take-home message about burnout: it doesn't have to become chronic or to recur, but you will need to make timely and significant changes to prevent that happening.

Burnout is a process that people have been observed to travel through over time. Although there is a range of different models, the most widely known is that by Christina Maslach and colleagues, who suggest that burnout has three components or stages: exhaustion, cynicism or depersonalisation, and a sense of ineffectiveness or diminished accomplishment. Any of these symptoms indicates that something is out of balance and needs to be changed. Most of us don't initially know what to look for, though, and find ourselves moving through the stages. Early on, often after being under considerable pressure for an extended period, people report feeling tired and also anxious in a way that does not settle over the weekend. They commonly report sleeping poorly on Sunday nights and experiencing physical symptoms of anxiety when getting ready for work on Mondays. If these early signs go unaddressed and the pressures continue, some people find themselves having discontented and even cynical thoughts about their workplace. Eventually, if exhaustion, dissatisfaction, and the original pressures continue unabated, some people find that the quality of their work suffers and that as a result they have lower regard for themselves and an even lower regard for the workplace. This experience is often made worse by the behaviour of colleagues, and especially by unsupportive behaviour when we expected more or better. At this point, people can often also feel anxious about their job security. If a person who is in this situation is unable to get a break or make major changes to their situation, they are at increased risk of moving from burnout to a form of chronic stress, or an anxiety or mood disorder. It is certainly not inevitable that the process of burnout will lead to a diagnoseable mental health condition, but it is certainly a risk. In some countries there are higher rates of depression and suicide among a number of the professions that contribute to the ranks of therapists, medical doctors and psychologists among them. More common is the lasting impact on how a person thinks about themselves and their competence to do their job and about their work sector. As burnout is particularly common among people who work with people, and people who were originally idealistic about work and motivated to do their roles from a desire to help others, this impact on self-confidence and self-regard in helping can be particularly devastating.

In his recent book, *The End of Burnout: Why work drains us and how to build better lives* (2022), Jonathan Malesic builds on the work by Maslach and colleagues, which suggests that the origins of burnout are in the gaps between our expectations and the reality of our work. He posits that that gap has become even wider as US culture, and all of us who are influenced by it, have come to think of work and working hard as not just about earning an income but proving our value, giving us dignity, and providing us a sense of meaning and opportunity for growth. Perhaps as an attempt to improve the quality of work, staff have been asked to give more emotionally at work, but without commensurate financial reward. Because these attitudes and trends are so widespread, managers themselves take them for granted and are often unaware of the deep human impact of work, and especially work with people. While acknowledging the importance of improving pay and conditions, Malesic is wary of these shifts if they become another reason to expect longer hours and increased commitment from workers. He suggests instead that the remedy for the ubiquity of burnout culture is in a shift that values workers rather than the work. At an individual level, he argues that the burnout pattern can only be broken as workers reconsider their own material expectations, reduce work where possible, and use their free time to nurture their inner needs and life beyond work.

This move is easier said than done, though. As I have mentioned to colleagues Malesic's thesis—that we have come to believe that work and working hard are not just about earning an income but that they prove our value, give us dignity, and provide a sense of meaning and opportunity for growth—I have been startled by their responses. Almost universally, these elements have been acknowledged as true in their experience, and as positive. We have absorbed these messages very deeply. At present, our understanding of the risks is comparatively superficial.

Suggestions

The best way to deal with burnout is to avoid it and to respond to stress early.

If you are noticing some warning signs, look up the Maslach Burnout Inventory. You might also look up resources around self-care and avoiding burnout on the website of your professional body.

If you can intervene early in the process, then strategically cutting back your client numbers or days can often prevent burnout developing, even when there are considerable challenges in the workplace.

Some people avoid burnout by making a big change: a new job, further study, extra responsibility, significant changes in work-life balance, a long holiday or a new therapy.

Burnout seems to arise in situations where there is a chronic imbalance between what is expected from a person and the resources that person has available to support them in their role. Consider if there is anything you can do to alter the balance of expectations and resources in your role. This may include changing your own expectations about yourself and what the work can realistically offer you and your clients.

If you are exhibiting all three signs of burnout, it is likely that nothing short of a radical change will reverse the process. Rarely, an employer offers their staff member a transfer into a different role. Sometimes, an employer is willing to restructure work and provide additional resources in a timely way. Sometimes, an employer is willing to let someone go on stress-leave for a period. These are all options you might consider. In the spirit of honesty, though, in my observation many people who take such leave don't return to their roles. The difference between how they feel in and out of the job speaks for itself and they find ways of moving elsewhere.

If you have experienced burnout once, you may have an increased risk of experiencing it again. This may be related to our underlying thoughts, rules, and assumptions, including those that brought us to therapy work in the first place and that potentially drive us in ways that are problematic. Some of these may be unique to us and our backgrounds. Others may be absorbed from our wider culture, including those mentioned by Jonathan Malesic, that our worth comes from our work and working hard, and that work is a place where we can fully express and live into our values. In addition, of course, our previous experience of burnout may have reinforced ways of thinking about ourselves and others, our work, and the world, that place us at increased risk. These might include the beliefs that others have lower standards than ourselves, that we are often misunderstood, or that workplaces or managers don't really care for clients but are focused on things like the financial bottom line. If you find yourself heading toward what feels like a second or third experience of burnout, take a break and give some serious thought to what you might be bringing to your work that contributes to your vulnerability.

One of the most powerful tools I know for preventing burnout is an idea called 'extreme self-care.' In Chapter 12 of their book, *Therapist as Life Coach: Transform your practice* (2002), on self-care, Patrick Williams and Deborah Davis advise life coaches to treat themselves regularly to what they might previously have thought of as a luxury. They describe this is 'out-of-the-normal, regular, high-quality self-care.' Examples could include a month-long holiday each year to somewhere you really want to go, a day off each month, a get-away every three months, regular massages, weekly manicures, and so on. This level of self-care also includes developing positive daily rituals. Examples they give include meditation and journal writing or other activities that help you connect with your spiritual self. We will return to the idea of spiritual resources in the next chapter. For now, though, let me put the challenge to you that longevity in your work as a therapist may require a level of self-care that feels like an indulgence to you at present. I encourage you to live into this suggestion and see if it is true for you. I suspect that one of the reasons this level of self-care is effective is that it begins to shift our relationship to our work in some of the ways suggested by Jonathan Malesic, where we expect somewhat less from our work, and invest more in our life beyond work.

As I noted above, however, it is very hard for most of us to expect less from our work. Sometimes parents manage this when they have young children; but perhaps more often they are torn between valuing the role of child-rearing and all that society has told them, and that they personally believe, about the importance of work. If after reading this section, or your own brush with burnout, you are beginning to contemplate a different relationship to work, I would encourage you to consider a review of your values. In my experience, therapists divide clearly into those who know about values inventories, reviews and their uses, and those who do not. If you are in the first category, you will know where to find a values inventory and may even have a working draft of your own. If this is new territory for you, I recommend the chapters about values in *The Happiness Trap* (2008), by Russ Harris. Harris suggests that a values review consider at least the following domains:

- family relationships
- marriage, couple and intimate relationships
- parenting
- friendships and social life
- career and employment
- education, personal growth and development
- recreation, fun and leisure
- spirituality

- citizenship, environment and community life, and
- health and physical well-being.

Feel free to add any other domains that seem important to you. Then prepare the questions that you might like to ask yourself, keeping in mind that values are about things that are of ongoing importance to you rather than goals that can be achieved and ticked off your list once and for all. Harris suggests such questions as, 'What is important to me in this domain?', 'What qualities do I want to bring to this relationship/situation?' and 'What behaviour and activities would I like to be doing/sharing in this relationship/situation?'

Such a values inventory can serve many purposes. My reason for suggesting it here is to support you to see your values around career and employment in the context of your other values. While work may help us to live according to our values in other domains, it is just possible that aspects of our work, or the way it affects us, may be detrimental to other values. It can be helpful to acknowledge those tensions if you are contemplating changing your relationship to work. In addition, it may be that values in some of these other domains, provide ways to hold work differently. For example, spiritual values might shape how you understand what you are doing at work, so it is less about you and your dignity and worth and more about service to others or God. Or perhaps values in other areas such as health or relationships reveal themselves as so important that your expectations about work and what it can offer reduce and rearrange themselves accordingly.

Workplace Tips

If you are in a position to influence decision-making in your workplace, be alert to both the client load and type of client that workers are carrying. Do what you can to contain daily client loads, increase the variety of client loads, factor in sufficient administrative time, and prioritise breaks and refreshing opportunities for professional development training.

Take-home message:

We should expect and prepare for crises in our relationship to our work. Even when some of the more common crises occur, with timely action it is possible to recover and thrive. Be prepared for the possibility, though, that such crises may require significant changes on your part, from a new job to a new perspective on what is important to you.

Where to next?

We consider a further type of professional crisis, the crisis of faith in therapy itself.

CHAPTER 7

Crises of Faith

In this second chapter on professional crises let us return briefly to the parallel with couple crises introduced in the previous chapter. You may recall the idea that couples who stay together will face at least five crises in their relationship, and my suggestion that something similar may be true if we are to continue our work as therapists. I think this parallel can be extended further. In order to stay together, couples have to find ways of negotiating crises. If in addition to surviving, they want their relationship to remain alive and to become stronger in the process, they each need to grow, and find ways of doing so fruitfully alongside the other. To do this, they need to reflect on and communicate about the sensitive places that exist in any long-term human relationship. In the case of professional crises, at such times of stretching and growth, a big change may be what's needed: a new job, further study, extra responsibility, significant changes in our work-life balance, a long holiday or a new therapy. At other times, some significant reflection may be required. Nowhere is this truer than for professional crises of faith. These are, in fact, the crises that gave this book its title, the ones that may produce outright disenchantment.

We have touched on several sources of such crises in this book. For example, people experiencing burnout sometimes feel they can no longer work in an organisation or an industry. The experience suggests to them that the organisation or industry is unworkable as it is. Many of the professionals who are resigning or retiring early in the wake of the COVID-19 pandemic are doing so for these reasons. As well, or alternatively, they may form the conclusion that the workplace or industry is not good for them, or that they are ill-suited to the work or even positively harmful to clients. That particular crisis—one of self-doubt—often also arises from longstanding ways of being in the world, including self-sacrificing or high standards patterns.

> *If my work is not appreciated, I might as well leave.*
> *If I can't do this to my standards, I can do something else instead.*

And, of course, high standards may also fuel discontent and disappointment with workplaces and organisations.

Other crises of faith are triggered by slow and hard work with clients. Thoughts may include, I'm making no difference ... I'm not helping... I can't do therapy ... some people (most of my clients) are too damaged to be helped, and so on.

For some therapists crises of faith relate to disappointments with particular therapies. While CBT is my primary therapy of choice, I have a colleague of psychodynamic persuasion who calls it Cold Barren Therapy. I tell myself that such critics have never really delved into the therapy or experienced the power it has over such a wide range of issues. That said, after so many years working with it, I recognise its limits. Having experienced the impact of experiential chair-work in Schema Therapy, I can see that engaging clients with the emotional origins of their thinking and life patterns shifts things at a greater speed and depth than CBT. In addition, if the client does have very difficult life circumstances, evaluating thoughts sometimes shows them to be true. The Defusion strategies from ACT may be more helpful. If they have trauma symptoms at a level that makes it hard to concentrate or organise themselves, they find it even more difficult than the average client to complete take-home tasks. If they have literacy difficulties, CBT may only ever be useful in modified form, and something like Eye Movement Desensitisation and Reprocessing (EMDR) may be needed. Now none of these limitations take away my appreciation for CBT. It is very powerful in its place. My experience is not unique in this regard. Many experienced therapists, whatever their first love or first training in therapy, discover with time the limits of that modality. With that often comes the temptation to let go of a therapy or drift from canonical application.

These last two very common options raise other problems for our belief in what we are doing as therapists. Despite the common self-perception among therapists that we become more skilled and effective with time, the relationship between years of experience and clinical expertise is one of many areas where there is little conclusive research evidence available. There are, in fact, some studies showing that newly graduated therapists are statistically more effective than more established therapists. One interpretation, at least, is that they are delivering therapies as they were intended to be delivered. This poses a conundrum for therapists who drift from canonical delivery of therapy. We may think we are making better connection with our clients, but are we being self-deceiving? Very few of us do follow-up research with clients.

Other doubts still may assail us. A clinical supervisor once told me, 'I think that as long as a therapist believes in a treatment approach, clients engage with it and get better'. Now this may be a further explanation for the good outcomes of beginning therapists, but what does this mean for our effectiveness as therapists if we begin to doubt the efficacy of our therapies?

The question of therapy efficacy is an important one in professional work where there is so much emphasis on 'evidence-based therapy' and so much dispute between therapists about the bar that has to be met for something to be 'evidence-based'. It is easy enough, based on one study, to declare an approach 'evidence-based'. If we place our confidence in higher standards of evidence, we need to acknowledge the difficulty of doing randomised, double-blind, placebo-controlled trials with many of our therapies, the very many poorly designed therapy trials that are conducted, and the very significant role of expectancy in trial outcomes, as well as the low rates of reproducibility for psychological studies. Most published intervention trials do find some improvement and most of the improvement is about non-specific factors like expectancy, engagement, and the relationship, rather than the therapy itself, the difference in efficacy between therapies, if any, being very small indeed. It's all enough to make you wonder if anything works. Worse still, knowing that much of the effect of therapy is in the therapeutic relationship, when our clients don't get better, we may find ourselves with no one left to blame but our clients or ourselves.

This type of crisis of faith is particularly relevant for work with clients with complex presentations who stabilise but at a level where they remain deeply depressed, prone to crises themselves, and persistently anxious. Or where, despite treatment for trauma and long-term patterns, they continue to be highly reactive, in conflict with those around them, or intermittently at risk of suicide. They do not feel like success stories. They keep coming but shift very little. General family medical practitioners work regularly with patients with such chronic conditions, but perhaps they are prepared for this in their training. Psychological training as I experienced it did not prepare me for clients who remain with a high degree of symptoms, despite my best efforts.

Before considering some suggestions, let us revisit some of the ideas from Jonathan Malesic about burnout in the previous chapter. You may notice that all the crises of faith outlined here in one way or another reflect a gap between our hopes for our work—to make a positive difference for our clients and to feel good about ourselves in the process—and what we experience. Any of these doubts could be the seeds of burnout. For those of us who have worked out ways of avoiding frank burnout, they are often material for disenchantment. For therapists where they have seen their work as a calling or vocation, that is, as a way they can bring their capacities to the needs of the world, these crises of faith may represent more than a gap between our hopes for work and what we experience. For example, if I have believed that given enough time and care I can help anyone or that anyone can experience healing, sufficient discouragement in the work may also be material for disillusionment with myself, others and the world more broadly.

Suggestions

Gratitude and appreciation

There are many hard aspects to our work as therapists, but there are also very many satisfactions. Few roles consistently involve such meaningful interpersonal connection. We are regularly privy to the most intimate parts of our clients' lives, as well as to the ways that small shifts in perspective can be transformative. If you are struggling with a crisis of faith, I recommend that you start with a one-off practice of gratitude for all the good things about your experience of work as a therapist. That may be enough to get you 'unstuck'. The best research we have on gratitude says that it only continues to be effective if it is used regularly. So, if you find that first practice helpful, consider how you might develop a gratitude habit associated with your work.

Follow-up research

At least in some settings, one way to assess your effectiveness is to use pre- and post-psychometric tests, wellbeing measures, or other client satisfaction and outcome ratings. Although this can be time consuming and confronting, if it is possible then this is one of the most straightforward ways of monitoring client progress, assessing your overall effectiveness, and making informed adjustments to your practice.

Redefine your work and success

You may recall the suggestion from 'Chapter 3: When the Work is Hard and Slow' that rather than seeing our work as primarily symptom-relief and rather than solely measuring our success by symptom-measures, it might be appropriate with some clients at least to reconsider our aims and how we define success. Perhaps it might support your work to use a bio-psycho-socio-spiritual assessment to guide treatment goals and then to review progress? Perhaps, in addition, you might consider an assessment and review that includes the role of society, culture, community, politics, and the environment? A client's symptom level may not have changed much, but have they experienced positive changes in other aspects of their lives?

It can also be helpful to consider a client's criteria for success. Remind yourself, if you can, clients more or less managed before they came to us, they somehow manage between sessions, and most of them will more or less manage without us—they have somehow found ways of functioning. We need to remember that what may well seem dysfunctional or terrible to us may be almost normal for our clients. This does not mean that we won't try to help and support, but only that our client's idea of success in therapy may be quite different from our own. There is a place for some questions from Solution Focussed Therapy:

What is the main problem you wish to get help with?
How important is it to you to get help with this problem?
What would change look like?
How would we know if we had made progress?
How confident do you feel about therapy helping you to change this problem?

Hope and trust

Hope and trust are relevant for both our clients and ourselves. Consider noticing, asking about, and nurturing a client's strengths. Their life circumstances and symptoms may be very challenging, but if as a result of our work they are more in touch with their inner resources, this may make a significant difference to how they feel about and approach these challenges.

A similar shift in perspective can also make a difference for therapists. When I was working for Quit Victoria, we were told that the average person had around fifteen attempts to stop smoking before they stopped for good. When we are talking on the phone to people who were seeking to stop smoking, we all knew that this was not likely to be their last attempt. We also knew that to eventually get to the place where they stopped smoking forever, they would need skills, knowledge, and encouragement to gradually address all the barriers to cessation in their lives. We might not see the final successful outcome, but we were contributing to that outcome. This is true more broadly for our work as therapists. Much of the time we don't know where our work fits in the context of our client's life. Our hope is at very least to do no harm, but ideally to support them a little further on their journey, whether that is through a particular crisis or toward a somewhat richer, fuller, and more meaningful life, to borrow a phrase from Russ Harris, author of *The Happiness Trap*.

Value what you do

Sometimes though, the circumstances of a person's life make it hard to trust that we have contributed positively, whether by the standards of the medical model, the bio-psycho-socio-spiritual model, or any other measure. Sometimes, as well, our clients have deeply entrenched ways of being or they are in the last few decades of life. In that situation, remind yourself of your values for work, for day-to-day human interactions, and for the community. Genuine, empathic engagement is better for your client and the community than none, and some human engagement is better for that person than isolation. This perspective requires humility, however, as this is a very modest goal and as a therapist it may not feel like what you signed up for: it is a far smaller but more foundational thing, this slow journeying alongside someone and gradual construction of human engagement. One therapist told me,

> I am thinking of my work with Sam. After four years, it didn't seem to me that we were making progress or that I had anything more to offer. He was also restless, although partly this was because he knew that for things to change he needed to make changes. And that was hard. I suggested to Sam and his mother that he consider a specialist referral to address specific issues. At first Sam's mother hesitated. She said, 'At very least your work makes a difference to me. He is more settled for a day or two after he sees you'. If I had not had this conversation with her, I would not have guessed. Sam certainly didn't tell me.

Of course, there are clients who are so unwell that they may not even seem to benefit from human contact. They may even seem agitated by it. In that situation, the act of turning up and being humane to another person is a little like the act of prayer in desperate circumstances. We offer it up anyway, because it is a response that we know and it is doing no harm, and because it feels like all we have. Maybe, at very least, like prayer, it may change the one who prays.

Acceptance and grief

Sitting in this place with clients affords at least two things. If I find myself wishing better for this client whose situation is so difficult, and if I can notice the wish, rather than fight against it or in some way attempt one more solution, perhaps I might come to some sort of acceptance, not liking or wanting their situation or mine, but allowing this terrible situation be, then maybe, just maybe, that holding may help the client. Sometimes, a client will shift, first into a deeper appreciation of their situation, and then into the truth that it will not change unless they think or do something differently. If I allow myself to accept and feel the pain of this situation, rather than fighting with it and adding to my own suffering as a therapist, I may model this option to my client. Perhaps if I can acknowledge the pain of this situation, if not to the client than to myself, I can grieve for the client. We may support the client to grieve but if they don't have insight enough or yet, we may need to let ourselves grieve. It is too little recognised how much grieving therapists do for their clients but also, if we acknowledge it, for our communities and aspects of our world. Although we work with individuals, when you have seen enough clients, it is possible to see patterns and to discern at that bigger level the many gaps between how we would like things to be and how things are. Jewish scripture has in it lament Psalms or songs that may be read individually but are very often meant to be read collectively. One of the very hard aspects of therapeutic work is that practitioners are often solitary as well as very diverse in our practice. It is difficult to find places for collective lament. If you can, find peers with whom you can have these conversations and caring others who are able to lament with you, or at very least, who can tolerate hearing your lament.

A change of heart

Individually or collectively, though, this sort of sitting with pain and grief does often shape convictions. For me, this includes a growing conviction about the care that we need to give children. Perhaps the hard parts of your work shape in you other convictions. Perhaps such convictions also shape in us action. In many professional bodies, there are interest groups and like-minded individuals wanting to see change or animated by ideas about what might support change. There is advocacy going on at many levels. It may be that some such action is calling to you as a response to your own pain, grief, and disenchantment.

Recognising the spiritual dimension to your work

My mention of prayer earlier hints at another set of resources you may draw on—spiritual ones. It is interesting, for research coming out of secular universities and reported by secular organisations, how consistently the literature on self-care now mentions the need to attend to the spiritual domain. None of this very clearly defines 'spiritual', but I take this to mean whatever a person understands as their deepest inner and outer resources. One definition of spirituality that I've found helpful is that by Solution-Oriented therapist Bill O'Hanlon in his book, *Pathways to Spirituality: Connection, wholeness, and possibility for therapist and client* (2006). There he defines spirituality as connection, compassion, and contribution, and identifies the following areas of connection:

- to the soul, the deeper self, the spirit,
- to or through the body,
- to another being,
- to community,
- through nature,
- by participating in, creating, or appreciating art, and
- to the Universe, Higher Power, God, or Cosmic Consciousness.

It is a helpful model for us as therapists to consider areas we are neglecting in our own self-care and connection. We will return to this consideration in our final chapter. It is also a useful framework within which to listen for our clients' experiences of disconnection, and nurture their paths to reconnection.

One of the reasons that therapists need to take spiritual resources seriously is the often-unacknowledged spiritual aspect to the work with clients. This won't be a surprise to pastoral workers and clergy reading this book, but many of us will not have made this link before. If spirituality and wholeness is characterised by connection, compassion, and contribution, including connection across the earlier mentioned domains, when clients are struggling in these areas, this is often because they have experienced what could be thought of as a spiritual injury. With a primarily secular audience in mind, I could restate that in the following way: if we as humans were made for connection, or at very least seem to work best when we have it, then profound ruptures in connection wound us at this deepest level for which we struggle to find agreed secular language. When we are working with clients with complex presentations and those who struggle to make change, we are observing and in the presence of this wounding, whether to their sense of self, their relationship to their bodies, their relationship with others, their engagement with all the good things or this world, or their sense of meaning, values, and ultimate context.

With this in mind, and although this is a long way from how many of us might see ourselves as therapists, there is an aspect of the secular priest to our roles as therapists, as we work toward the healing of connections. Earlier communities recognised this in our forebears—the shamans, medicine men, wise women, and healers. They understood that these were liminal roles, standing somewhere between here and another world, the known and the unknown.

It's important to own the importance of what therapists are about when they are working at these deeper levels of connection with clients. In Mahayana Buddhism there are the Bodhisattvas, people who have reached enlightenment and who could go to nirvana but who choose to stay to hold the whole suffering world in compassion until all can reach enlightenment. In Christianity, Jesus's care to others involved healing both physical and mental ailments. Incidentally, his commitment to getting away for quiet times and for prayer is a singularly powerful model of our need to attend to self-care and to enlivening resources. In Christianity, in addition, Jesus is understood as somehow bearing to God all the hurts people do to themselves and to others or have had done to them, in a way that brings about forgiveness and healing. Of course, the Bodhisattvas have to their advantage in their task that they have achieved enlightenment, and in Christian belief, Jesus is God's son, both human and divine. While learning a great deal about life and love over time, we therapists are thoroughly human. Holding the suffering and pain of the world with compassion, and bearing the hurts of world with the possibility of forgiveness and healing is very hard work, even if we are only doing this for our small set of clients, and only sharing in these tasks as pale reflections of the healing archetypes captured in these traditions. And while adherents of these traditions may draw some comfort that they are participating in the spirit of these actions, we need also to hold in mind the impact on us of this work. I recall what Hildegard of Bingen says in one of her letters, possibly as a result of her persistent migraines: 'Those who long to complete God's work must always bear in mind that they are fragile vessels, for they are only human'. Put practically, expect this work to have a significant impact on your mind, body, and spirit. Even if you want to be the perfect therapist, you are not God and trying to act like God without God's resources will not be good for you.

If you are doing spiritual work, supporting people at the deep level of their connections, you need spiritual resources, including nurturing your own connections. I urge you to draw deeply on the lifegiving spiritual connections and resources that you have available to you. This may include practices that connect you to your deeper inner self, to your body, to others, to all the good things of earth, and to your values, sense of meaning, and ultimate context, including but not limited to your religious beliefs and practices.

Workplace Tip

If you are in a position to influence decision-making in your workplace, do what you can to acknowledge these harder aspects of client work. This sort of acknowledgement might propel initiatives to nurture team cohesion and peer support, resource staff wellbeing champions, or build a staff self-care library.

Take-home message:

Crises of faith are coming if you remain a therapist. Be prepared to journey through them, to engage in significant reflection, and to consider the opportunities there for growth and going deeper in your work and your experience of life.

Where to next?

Having taken this deep dive, let's get back to the basics of self-care in the final chapter.

Chapter 8

In Conclusion: Back to—Self-Care—Basics

Welcome to the final chapter of *The Disenchanted Therapist*. I'm glad you made it. In the Introduction, I said that I was assuming that if you were having struggles with therapist disenchantment:

- you had already set aside time to reflect on how your own thoughts and long-term ways of being in the world were contributing to the situation,
- you were intentionally using all the therapeutic strategies and skills you had available,
- you were discussing your work with a professional, competent, and wise therapist-colleague who was acting as your clinical supervisor or peer mentor,
- you were regularly planning and engaging in professional development learning that was relevant to the struggles you were experiencing, and that
- you were establishing a personal and professional discipline of intentional self-care.

In a conversation about this book with a friend who is a theologian, he said, 'Talking about self-care to therapists can't be easy. A bit like commending prayer and Bible study to us theologians. We know full well we need them, but it feels hard because we are immersed in this material all day.' He is right, of course. This daily contact with messages about self-care—including those we deliver—is one of many reasons that it can be difficult for us therapists to intentionally implement our own self-care. At this point, now that you have a clearer sense of the issues that might be contributing to your own experience of therapist disenchantment, let's return to that list with a more focussed appreciation of its importance. Here are some thoughts about how to begin, return to, or recover these practices, including a summary of some of the growth suggestions that appear in earlier chapters.

You will notice that there is considerable overlap between these essentials. For example, reflecting on your situation is likely to suggest which therapy strategies, self-care or professional development you might need. Let this encourage you. Any time and energy you commit to these essentials will pay dividends. It also suggests the importance of reflection. Let's begin there.

Reflection

You need more than self-care as it is often superficially defined. You need a practice of reflection into your own inner processes. We noted earlier that there is a huge risk for therapy students and practitioners who want to do this work without growing deeper in our knowledge of ourselves and our ability to work with that content.

When people are learning to meditate with an instructor, one of the early recommendations is that they start a meditation journal. This is thought of as a space for noting down how the meditation went, including what arose for the person during the meditation. As well, though, the journal provides a space to intentionally begin the process of self-reflection, generally, and to apply it to an emerging discipline of meditation, specifically.

If you don't already have one, I recommend that you commence a therapy journal. Our days are full, I know, but if you want to become very good at something, be that being a partner, parent or therapist, some regular reflection helps. For one thing, it may highlight issues to take to clinical supervision. As well, if you notice yourself avoiding your journal, that may suggest there are some things bubbling away that need your time and attention.

I have included here some reflection questions for after client sessions. You will notice that the questions are in four groups: questions for noticing patterns related to our history and to possible transference and countertransference, some standard debriefing questions, questions about additional resources, and then questions about client strengths. If this list speaks to you, I encourage you to make it your own and modify it to your needs. Over time, you probably won't need to answer each question for each client. In fact, it's unlikely you will have the time to do so! But reviewing the list at the end of a session or in preparation for clinical supervision is likely to highlight some ways forward that you didn't consider in the moment.

Reflective questions:

Noticing
What did I notice about the client's responses and my own? Where were there strong emotions, changes in emotional tone, places of frustration, and responses that felt familiar?

Debriefing
What went well in the session?
What could I improve on?
Was I sufficiently prepared?
How can I prepare for my next session with this client?
Did the session highlight any gaps in my knowledge and skills?
If so, how can I address that gap? Do I own resources on this topic or does my professional body have resources on this topic?

Other resources
Are there other specialised or additional counselling or psychological services that this client would be eligible to receive? (For example, counselling specifically for financial guidance, family violence, carer issues, road or work accidents, drug and alcohol concerns, or victims of crime supports, etc.)

Are there generic resources such as problem solving, stress management etc., that might be useful to this client?

Is there psychological information on depression, anxiety etc., which might be useful to this client?

Are there any other supports or services that might be relevant? (bibliotherapy; e-mental health; material aid; community groups and activities; financial compensation)

Client strengths
What are the supports in this person's life?
What are the strengths in this person's story?
Where is there life, love, light, and freedom in this story?

Therapeutic strategies and skills

One of the great benefits of being therapists is that we specialise in thinking about and supporting human reflection, motivation, and change. This is also a downside, because it is hard to ignore the many places in our lives where we are not taking our own advice. This is human, of course, and we need to be kind to ourselves about this, as well as clear-sighted.

You may have noticed that in this book I have been systematically drawing on the therapy strategies and skills known to me. I've been doing that because these are the resources at my disposal when I think about how to support myself in the work of being a therapist. As therapists are a very broad group with many different theoretical orientations and frames of reference, please take what is useful to you from this book and discard the rest. Start with what is familiar to you, and consider how you can intentionally use those ideas to support yourself as you tackle the roots of your disenchantment. As I've said elsewhere, any time you take to acquire new skills and strategies is a worthwhile investment.

Clinical supervision

I have attended at least monthly clinical supervision across each year of my work as a psychologist. For four of those years, as I was undertaking further training, I attended supervision fortnightly or more often. Clinical supervision is foundational for me. While there is a great deal that we can learn from formal training, the nature of our work requires apprenticeship, that is, supervised practice on the job. As well, the very private nature of our work requires some sort of regular reflection and scrutiny to ensure both quality and safety. The regular parade of therapists called to account for inappropriate practices and boundary violations including but not limited to sexual misconduct, attests to how easy it is for us to be self-deceiving. This is one of many reasons that increasing numbers of professions and workplaces also insist on that bare minimum of monthly clinical supervision.

So, if you are dissatisfied with the relationship you have with your clinical supervisor, address it with them, or find someone else. Perhaps there are ways in which you could make the supervision you have more effective, either by negotiation with your clinical supervisor or a shift in your attitude to the space, or a combination of these. For further ideas, see Chapter Four of Hawkins and Shohet, on 'Being an effective supervisee'. If your workplace is providing management supervision but not clinical supervision of your client-based work, ask for such supervision. If it can't be provided, then find a way to obtain it. Your life as a therapist depends on it.

You may remember that in Chapter 6, I recommended that you arrange extra clinical supervision whenever you need it, whether this is related to particular client cases or when starting a new role or increasing hours, or when you are experiencing one of the forms of personal or professional crisis we touched on in that Chapter and the next.

The cost of clinical supervision is the most frequent barrier for therapists. If you need clinical supervision in order to complete your qualification, some workplaces will provide it for you as part of your employment. This was certainly a consideration for me when I was looking for work after graduation. Keeping that cost in mind, it will help if you can approach the idea of clinical supervision with some flexibility. Perhaps your professional body or workplace offers free peer-supervision groups? If they don't, perhaps you could start a group? Or perhaps you have a more experienced colleague who would be happy to meet with you once a month if they could claim it as an hour of professional development for themselves. They might be able to make that argument if the topic of your supervision or practice as a supervisor is part of their own professional development plan. Get as much clinical supervision as you can, as often as you can, from a combination of sources.

If you find a clinical supervisor or supervision group that works for you, stay in that arrangement. An experienced colleague of mine mentioned that he had been in a workplace peer-supervision group for many years, and that over time the group had developed a very collegial and supportive tone. The individuals in it had come to trust each other and the space. This had been very important for him, he said, when recently he had experienced a professional embarrassment. This was a safe place where he could share the experience and receive support. We need these places as therapists. Do what you can to nurture your own support network.

Professional development

My professional body expects that its members will create a professional development plan and then review it every year, and that they will complete a certain number of hours of professional development every year. This is a fine example of a professional expectation and process that can seem burdensome but that is actually a way of codifying something that is essential to professional practice. We need to refresh, refine, and add to our skills, throughout our careers, but with particular intention at the beginning and towards the end. This is important for us and our energy for the work. It is also important for our clients.

You may recall that in the course of this book I have made several specific suggestions about professional development training. The first, in Chapter 3, 'When the Work is Hard and Slow,' was that as soon as possible and then from time to time in your career, you read and do courses on how to respond to suicide. The second, in Chapter 6, and the section 'Too Much Too Soon,' was that you start by becoming very good at your core therapy. The third, also in that chapter, was that in advance of any professional crisis, you know your code of ethics, and the relevant legislation around your work. I suggested that you keep this area on your list of potential professional development activities, even if only in the form of some occasional reading.

Very quickly, your clients will prompt you to think about further professional development. They will be constantly arriving with issues and concerns where you need additional skills. As an example, I have recently been completing further training regarding sleep. This is very relevant to my work as almost every client either has had or currently has sleep difficulties. Of course, the list of things you could know is almost endless and may feel dispiriting. While I encourage you to add to your professional development plan a wish-list for future professional development, attempt to think strategically as well about areas that you would like to develop in the short-to-medium term. Perhaps you are struggling in particular ways with your work? Is there training that might speak to that need? Make that a priority. Or perhaps you want to build skills for working with PTSD or complex trauma? Perhaps you need additional skills in cross-cultural competence? Perhaps the time has come for you to train as a clinical supervisor yourself?

Of course, for therapists, continuing professional development training often also includes study toward further formal qualifications. A colleague told me that a Masters in Couple Counselling and a PhD in Psychology, two further qualifications beyond his training in clinical psychology, were key experiences that helped to keep him in the profession over a forty-year period, each adding new skills and knowledge and giving him a boost of energy for his work.

The cost of professional development and further training is often a barrier, much as it is with clinical supervision, and especially for early-career therapists. If your workplace or local area public mental health service provides free or discounted professional development, keep an eye out for what they are offering. Perhaps your professional association provides listings of events, including occasional discounts? Take advantage of those opportunities. I schedule time to read my professional body's journals and magazines, and I record that as professional development time. I also regularly read books related to the therapies I use and the conditions I treat, and especially the ones where I sense a gap in my knowledge. There are now also increasing numbers of free high-quality materials online in the form of recorded webinars and podcasts.

Self-care

When I write about self-care as a personal and professional discipline, I am doing so intentionally. In a world that is leery of discipline, this can be a hard sell. The truth is, though, that to function well and consistently over time in any part of our life will require disciplines or practices of one sort of another. For therapists, self-care is one such discipline. This means that your self-care plan is either written down or can be summarised in a sentence or two, and that there are clear elements of self-care in how you arrange your day, your week, your month, and your year. The chances are that you already have some sort of self-care in place. I invite you to take this to the next level by documenting it and entering regular self-care commitments into your diary. Getting it down on paper will also highlight gaps. For example, I manage my daily self-care reasonably well, but I find it harder to prioritise a break once a month. I know that's important though, as such breaks often serve as something to look forward as week follows week.

You will recall the idea that a central contributor to burnout is an imbalance between the demands on you and the resources available to you. This suggests that our self-care plans, whether for emergency situations or for day-to-day use, may be made stronger by considering both those elements.

Demands

Start by considering your ideal daily number of clients. Reducing this number by even one or two may make the difference for you between a sense of pressure and poise. I had a colleague who went further than this and intentionally saw clients for only 45 minutes in each hour. Rather than running from session to session, this gave him time to prepare and write up notes, as well as a brief moment to catch his breath between clients. He found that this allowed him to see six or more clients daily without an accumulating sense of weariness. If you have the freedom to do so, you can also experiment with your ideal number of client-days across a week.

Another way to reduce demands is to be intentional about whether you will take referrals and when you refer to others. You may find that you have insufficient time to treat your current clients effectively, let alone to provide adequate care to new clients. In that circumstance, it may be appropriate to close your books for a time, and to direct incoming referrals to other practitioners. While there are some settings and times where no other therapists are available, in many places there is no shortage of alternative care, especially now in this age of online therapy and telehealth. You do not need to be all things to all people.

Similarly, try to be as clear as you can about the limits of your competence and how fresh your knowledge is about the issue or condition affecting the client. People come to therapists with a vast array of issues. Even if you advertise your specialties clearly, at least a proportion of the people who come to see you will need specialist treatment for something that you know little about. You may be delaying them getting the care they need if you unintentionally convey that you can treat something you can't. It is always best practice within a session or two to have a conversation with your client about your assessment and treatment plan. A client may be quite happy to commence more general work with you for a time, knowing that they will need to transfer to a specialist for that other issue at some point in the future. It will be your role to point out any costs and benefits of such a delay. It is important that you have their informed consent for your shared plan and the consequences of that plan.

Finally, a few words about the other demands in our life beside work. Sometimes, and in fact quite often, the demands of work look quite manageable but they occur in the context where a lot else is going on: we are juggling many other commitments and sometimes even a personal crisis or two. Sometimes work is the easiest thing to cut back. At other times, though, that income is essential and something else may need to give. These aren't easy changes to make or to negotiate with others, of course. One of the benefits of being a therapist, though, is that you probably know something about communication, problem-solving, finding solutions, and making decisions.

Resources

Scheduling a day or up to a week off temporarily reduces the demands you are experiencing and it provides an opportunity for refreshment. In that way, a break of any length helps on both sides of the demands-and-resources ledger.

What you do with your time off also matters. Sometimes, of course, rest and sleep are what is required. Much of the time, though, we will be nourished by particular activities. These may be forms of relaxation, meditation, prayer or journaling. They may be exercise or other activities we enjoy or value and that constitute a mental break from work. They may be smaller or larger luxuries or indulgences that both convey we are valuing ourselves and acknowledge the impact of our work. I refer you back to the idea of 'extreme self-care', and the invitation to plan 'out-of-the-normal, regular, high-quality self-care'. If you are looking for more ideas, your professional organisation is likely to have a section on practitioner self-help resources on their website. If what you have read here has sparked your interest in therapist self-care, I can recommend as further reading the comprehensive and evidenced-based book, Leaving It At The Office: A guide to psychotherapist self-care (2018), by John C. Norcross and Gary R. Vandenbos.

When you are thinking about what to include in your self-care plan, you might consider the areas of connection identified by Bill O'Hanlon and summarised in the previous chapter. How do you connect:

- to your soul, deeper self, spirit
- to or through your body
- to another being
- to community
- through nature
- by participating in, creating, or appreciating art, and
- to the Universe, Higher Power, God, or Cosmic Consciousness?

Perhaps you sense gaps in one or more of these areas of connection that you want to address in your self-care plan. This can be a powerful tool to assess and replenish your own resources.

Having finished the previous chapter encouraging you to attend to spiritual resources, let me return to that theme for a moment. If your work draws on particular resources, you will need to find ways to replenish those resources. If your work is with distressed families or disturbed children, spending time with supportive and functioning families, and happy and well-cared-for children, will be important. Sometimes, regular contact with colleagues who are passionate and energetic about supporting families and children can substitute for lifegiving contact with family. If you use a particular therapy or therapeutic orientation, you will benefit from continuing to read and complete high-quality professional development in that area. Much of it might be familiar to you, but you will be hearing again about its benefits from a fresh perspective, thereby renewing your energy for the work. If your work draws on faith or spiritual resources, you will need to find ways of replenishing those resources. Recent research on ministry burnout suggests that, more than anything else, a pastoral worker's relationship to God has to be nourished. Presumably this is also relevant for those of us whose workplace values are animated by religious and spiritual beliefs and practices. Verbal acknowledgement of these loyalties may not be sufficient as a resource.

There is a closely related invitation here. Getting really good at your work is a way of creating resources. It's true that it takes time, effort, and financial resources, initially and over time, but this is an example of a practice that more than repays any cost. When you know your therapy or treatment well, because you have returned to it again and again, reflecting on and adding to what you know, you will develop a level of skill for assessment and treatment that will have its own pleasures. You will know that this is happening when you have a sense of the right way to proceed with cases that would previously have been challenging, and when your clinical judgement proves to be correct.

As I mentioned in Chapter 5, 'Context is Everything,' there is another way of creating resources for yourself, and that is through developing processes and documents that serve your work with clients. When you take the time to digest what you need in order to practice well, and what your clients often need to take away from sessions, and then create or locate relevant tools, you are adding value to your work.

Finally, you will remember from Chapter 6 on professional crises that I urged you to build up support networks. The default in many places is that therapists either work alone or see their colleagues only when passing in the hallway, client in tow. It will need your commitment to work against the inertia in this pattern. Take the time to get to know the people you work with. Chat about your work. Learn about your colleagues as they talk about themselves and their work. Offer support where the need arises and practice asking for support. If you meet a colleague whom you respect, take opportunities to debrief and do what you can to keep in contact when one or either of you moves on to another role. Take whatever opportunities arise for group supervision. Consider joining professional interest groups of like-minded colleagues. If you are in a position to influence decision-making in your workplace, do what you can to encourage and facilitate these practices.

In addition to professional networks, do everything you can to build and maintain your personal networks of family, friends, acquaintances, and community. We were made for connections of all sorts, and we do best in community. This is as true for us as it is for our clients.

On this note, let us return to what brought you to this book in the first place. While not aiming to be comprehensive, my hope in writing this book was to help you spot, navigate, and overcome the common emotional challenges of client work, so that you can continue to love the work, effectively support clients, and grow professionally and personally. If you feel somewhat less alone and somewhat more resourced, my goal has been achieved. May your next encounter with therapist disenchantment be shorter but also more rewarding, as you emerge with a deeper understanding of yourself and greater confidence in your ability to weather the storms of this work. That said, this process of supporting ourselves and each other is one that continues. Before you close this book, I recommend that you return to any 'Suggestions' or 'Workplace Tips' that spoke to you. Make a note of them. In particular, if you noticed the urge to reach out for clinical supervision, or therapy, or some informal support, act on that urge.

Wishing you every good thing.

Reference List

Burns, D. (1989). *The Feeling Good Handbook*. New York: Harper-Collins Publishers.

Covey, S. R. (1989, 2004, 2020). *The 7 Habits of Highly Effective People: Powerful lessons in personal change*. New York, NY: Simon & Schuster.

Cozolino, L. (2004). *The Making of a Therapist: A practical guide for the inner journey*. New York & London: W. W. Norton & Company.

Jacob, G., van Genderen, H., & Seebauer, L. (2015). *Breaking Negative Thinking Patterns: A Schema Therapy self-help and support book*. Chichester & Oxford: Wiley Blackwell.

Hari, J. (2018). *Lost Connections: Uncovering the real causes of depression—and the unexpected solutions*. London et al.: Bloomsbury Circus.

Harris, R. (2007). *The Happiness Trap: Stop struggling, start living*. Dunedin, NZ & Gosford, NSW, Australia: Exisle Publishing.

Hawkins, P. & Shohet, R. (2006). *Supervision in the Helping Professions* (3rd ed.). Maidenhead, Berkshire & New York, NY: Open University Press and McGraw-Hill.

Herman, J. (1992). *Trauma and Recovery: The aftermath of violence—From domestic abuse to political terror*. New York: Basic Books.

Kellogg, S. (2015). *Transformational Chairwork: Using psychotherapeutic dialogues in clinical practice*. Lanham et al.: Rowman & Littlefield.

Malesic, J. (2022). *The End of Burnout: Why work drains us and how to build better lives*. Oakland, California: University of California Press.

Miller, W. R. & Rollnick, S. (1991). *Motivational Interviewing: Preparing people to change addictive behaviour*. New York & London: The Guilford Press.

Norcross, J. C. & Vandenbos, G. R. (2018). *Leaving It At the Office: A guide to psychotherapist self-care* (2nd ed.). New York and London: The Guilford Press.

O'Hanlon, B. (2006). *Pathways to Spirituality: Connection, wholeness, and possibility for therapist and client.* New York & London: W.W.

Norton & Company.

Phoenix Australia – Centre for Posttraumatic Mental Health and the Canadian Centre of Excellence – PTSD (2020). *Moral Stress Amongst Healthcare Workers During COVID-19: A Guide to Moral Injury*. Phoenix Australia – Centre for Posttraumatic Mental Health and the Canadian Centre of Excellence – PTSD, ISBN online: 978-0-646-82024-8.

Rothschild, B. (2023). *Help for the Helper: Preventing compassion fatigue and vicarious trauma in an ever-changing world* (2nd ed.). New York & London: W.W. Norton & Company.

Van Dernoot Lipsky, L. with Burk, C. (2009). *Trauma Stewardship: An everyday guide to caring for self while caring for others (illustrated edition)*. San Francisco, California: Berrett-Koehler Publishers.

Williams, P. & Davis, D. C. (2002). *Therapist as Life Coach: Transform your practice*, New York, NY: W.W. Norton Company, Inc.

Young, J. E. & Klosko, J. S. (1993). *Reinventing Your Life: The breakthrough program to end negative behaviour and feel great again.* New York, NY: Plume, Penguin Group.

Please consider leaving a review online.

Printed in Great Britain
by Amazon